SAGE was founded in 1965 by Sara Miller McCune to support the dissemination of usable knowledge by publishing innovative and high-quality research and teaching content. Today, we publish over 900 journals, including those of more than 400 learned societies, more than 800 new books per year, and a growing range of library products including archives, data, case studies, reports, and video. SAGE remains majority-owned by our founder, and after Sara's lifetime will become owned by a charitable trust that secures our continued independence.

Los Angeles | London | New Delhi | Singapore | Washington DC | Melbourne

KIDNEY TRANSPLANTS & SCAMS

KIDNEY TRANSPLANTS & SCAMS

INDIA'S TROUBLESOME LEGACY

Dr Ramesh Kumar

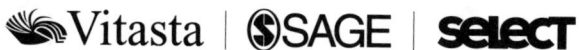

Los Angeles | London | New Delhi
Singapore | Washington DC | Melbourne

Copyright © Ramesh Kumar, 2020

All rights reserved. No part of this book may be reproduced or utilized in any form or by any means, electronic or mechanical, including photocopying, recording or by any information storage or retrieval system, without permission in writing from the publisher.

First published in 2020 by

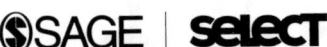 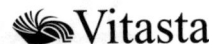

SAGE Publications India Pvt Ltd
B1/I-1 Mohan Cooperative Industrial Area
Mathura Road, New Delhi 110 044, India
www.sagepub.in

Vitasta Publishing Pvt Ltd
2/15 Ansari Road, Daryaganj
Delhi 110002
www.vitastapublishing.com

SAGE Publications Inc
2455 Teller Road
Thousand Oaks, California 91320, USA

SAGE Publications Ltd
1 Oliver's Yard, 55 City Road
London EC1Y 1SP, United Kingdom

SAGE Publications Asia-Pacific Pte Ltd
18 Cross Street #10-10/11/12
China Square Central
Singapore 048423

Published by Vivek Mehra for SAGE Publications India Pvt Ltd. Typeset in 11/16pt Georgia by Fidus Design Pvt. Ltd, Chandigarh.

Library of Congress Control Number: 2019954166

ISBN: 978-93-5388-234-1 (PB)

SAGE Vitasta Team: Manisha Mathews, Shruti Gupta, Papri Sri Raman and Anupama Krishnan

As a young doctor in the 1960s, I had watched the plight and misery of kidney failure patients helplessly. After fifty years, today these patients have hope for prolonging their lifespans, lead a healthier life, look after their young families, educate their children and live with hope.

I dedicate this book to my vast number of these fellow human beings with whom I was able to participate in their struggle to survive.

Thank you for choosing a SAGE product!
If you have any comment, observation or feedback,
I would like to personally hear from you.

Please write to me at **contactceo@sagepub.in**

Vivek Mehra, Managing Director and CEO, SAGE India.

Bulk Sales

SAGE India offers special discounts
for purchase of books in bulk.
We also make available special imprints
and excerpts from our books on demand.

For orders and enquiries, write to us at

Marketing Department
SAGE Publications India Pvt Ltd
B1/I-1, Mohan Cooperative Industrial Area
Mathura Road, Post Bag 7
New Delhi 110044, India

E-mail us at **marketing@sagepub.in**

Subscribe to our mailing list
Write to **marketing@sagepub.in**

This book is also available as an e-book.

CONTENTS

Foreword by Navin Chawla	ix
Flashback by Justice Sudershan Misra	xiii
A Word from My Heart	xv
Preface	xxi
My Blackened Face	xxv

Introduction	1
Cures and Costs	11
Pushing for an Organ Transplant Law	23
Kidney Transplant in India	33
Kidney Scams in India	39
India Becomes the World's Kidney Bazaar	49
Maximum City Mumbai Kidney Trade Epicentre	56
Kidney Racket in Tamil Nadu	70
Blood Donors, Drug Mafia, Dowry Kidneys in Kolkata	79
The Kidney King and the Great Escape	86
Kidney Scandal in Karnataka	100

CONTENTS

Tribals as Kidney Donors in Kerala	105
Horrifying Kidney Racket in Punjab	111
West Coast to the East	116
In the Heartland of MP, Bihar, UP	126
Kidney Scams in Delhi	131
Cyber Scams in Kidney Trade	165
Kidney Rackets Worldwide	173
The Human Element	180
Moving Forward	186
Epilogue	204
Appendix A	207
Appendix B	216
Appendix C	219
Acknowledgements	223
About the Author	229

FOREWORD

I read Dr Ramesh Kumar's narration of India's kidney racket with increasing despondency. An issue which was hitherto peripheral to my thinking has now become central to it. This is in major part because I have known Dr Kumar to be a medical practitioner not only of the highest competence (as evidenced, too, by his string of awards and accolades), but for his overwhelming integrity throughout his lifetime of healthcare delivery as a pioneering nephrologist and surgeon. In this book, he has exposed what many of us suspected: a well organised racket that trades on the susceptibilities of largely poor donors to benefit the rich. For these reasons, this first hand, authoritative and well documented book must be taken very seriously by our governments, administrators, judges and law makers, hospital proprietors and their managements, as well as law enforcing agencies, all of whom need to be made conscious of the deep malaise that exists in our midst.

The author holds that over 40 years ago, India earned the dubious distinction of the world's 'kidney bazaar'. Wealthy Indians as well as overseas visitors, (who converged here in the guise of 'medical tourists'), were attracted by the easy availability of body organs! This was especially so in the case of kidneys. In the West, there were strict laws and practices in place before a donor could donate an organ. India, on the other hand, had no law in place. It was only with the active support of Prime Minister Atal Bihari Vajpayee that a group of ethical pioneers in nephrology persuaded the government to pass much needed legislation to bring laws, guidelines and a system in place. However, as Dr Kumar's book tells us, there is still vast room for improvement. Illegal transplants continue to be carried out in 'underground' clinics and in some cases even in large well-known hospitals, where surgeons face a dilemma between trying to save lives often in the face of incomplete or overtly false paperwork.

It is saddening that poor 'donors' continue to be lured for a few thousand rupees into a twilight world of touts, false or dubious papers, fly-by-night medical centres, lax law agencies and unscrupulous doctors, all of whom are complicit when impoverished 'donors' are lured into selling their kidneys to non-relative recipients, in a nether world that has sprung up in practically every State, and more especially in the metros. This is one case where there is no distinction of caste, religion or nationality: there is just one line to be crossed here, that between the rich and the poor. I can sense Dr Kumar's anguish that this practice is going on even in well-known hospitals. He has not hesitated in naming some. He also brings to the fore true cases of exploitation; particularly sad is the exploitation of women, especially women relatives, who are often forced against their will to provide their kidney to their male relatives.

With a life-time of experience, Dr Kumar offers a solution. Road traffic victims are a source of harvesting of kidneys. This highlights the importance of organ donation from a cadaver source, which can save lives as well as avoid any form of exploitation. In India there are thousands of road accident victims every month. If their families would allow, these could be a source of much needed kidneys to save lives. For example, Delhi sees about seven or eight traffic fatalities a day. These could help save twice as many lives. This necessitates public awareness, which should begin. As the author reiterates, two kidneys save not just two lives but four, for this also renders free two dialysis machines, of which our country still has a great dearth.

The overwhelming lesson I take from this book is that it must both be widely read and also acted upon.

Navin Chawla
Former Chief Election Commissioner of India

FLASHBACK

I have observed Dr Ramesh Kumar closely for more than two decades as he shepherded the treatment of my wife, Smita, an accomplished lawyer, for renal failure and all that it entailed. From subcranial hematoma to dialysis to transplantation with all the ensuing consequences – he took care of it all and I must say, the more I saw, the greater my appreciation of the man and his skills.

In fact, with each passing year and the ever-present threat of her condition getting out of hand – as evidenced by one crisis after another linked to the malady, as all sufferers know, that may lead to a rapid collapse – you have a soar throat in the morning and you are in the ICU by midnight – Smita had developed a standard mantra, 'just get me to Doctor, he will set me right'. He did. Time and again. Until her last breath.

Such dedication does not come from professional degrees alone. It comes from rare qualities of the head and heart, both of which must be in sync and aligned in the right direction. It is because Dr Ramesh has these in great measure that he has been impelled to write this very insightful and compelling work on the seamier byproduct of the life-saving advances in kidney transplantation, and also bring to the fore the ethical conundrums faced by the medical profession. I cannot imagine any other leading expert of his stature, nor in any other field of expertise, undertaking such a venture, that too at the pinnacle of his highly successful career. This is because he genuinely cares, where others may be content to just rest on their laurels.

At a time when our society is undergoing major changes, not all of which are for the better and where, tragically and increasingly, even doctors and teachers have started praying to goddess Lakshmi, Dr Ramesh Kumar remains steadfast in his veneration of the goddess Saraswati, the goddess of learning, knowledge and wisdom. He himself is an icon who embodies Vishnu, the preserver, for all those who come in contact with him.

After having gone through the manuscript, I can only add that regardless of one's point of view on any of the different aspects covered by the author, one thing is clear – that henceforth, every meaningful discussion on the state of the law and practice of kidney transplantation in India must begin from this work.

Justice Sudershan Kumar Misra

A WORD FROM MY HEART

In those days, there used to be an imaginary dividing line on the road, today known as the Aurobindo Marg in Delhi, India's capital city. Even then, it was a very busy road leading to the airport in the south of the city. Facing south, at the junction were two of Delhi's most popular hospitals – the Safdarjung on the right and the All-India Institute of Medical Sciences (AIIMS) on the left. Road accidents were frequent on this road and the unwritten practice was – victims on the right of the divider would be taken to the Safdarjung Hospital and those on the left to AIIMS.

I am talking of the early 1980s and for a young kidney specialist, AIIMS was where one needed to be. Nephrology was an upcoming science and the department at the country's premier healthcare institution was also new and we at AIIMS took pride in providing the latest drugs and medicines available elsewhere in the world to our patients.

The use of intravenous cyclosporin drug was just beginning in England and United States; Sandoz (now Novartis) representatives offered the All India Institute of Medical Sciences a supply of Sandimune injections from the parent company in England. For all of us at AIIMS, the chance to work with branded cyclosporin was a very inspiring proposal.

In the nephrology department, a thirty-year-old young man was on haemo-dialysis[1] (also called hemodialysis or dialysis) with end-stage kidney failure. He urgently needed a kidney transplant. His younger brother was the only suitable member in the family who had volunteered to donate and became the prospective kidney donor, chosen by the doctors at AIIMS.

This young man was of similar blood group as the prospective recipient. The practice of 'tissue matching' had not begun. India had no particular rules and regulations at the time regarding organ donation.

It was decided that, at the operative procedure, the drug cyclosporin would be administered to the recipient brother. All arrangements with Sandoz in India and UK were completed to get the drug by the next flight to Delhi. The family was told of the arrangements and were requested to collect the consignment from Delhi airport at no cost.

Both the brothers were admitted in the hospital two days before the operation date. A day before the surgery, I received a frantic note from the duty nurse in the morning – that the 'donor' brother was missing from the bed and had himself gone to collect the medicine from the airport.

---

[1] This is a process of purifying the blood of a person whose kidneys are not working normally through an artificial membrane system.

We at once contacted the family. Two people – the recipient's wife and father – were available at the hospital. We were told that they did not have any other person with them to run around and get the medicine. Those were pre-mobile times, and this was quite a worrying period for all of us. There was no way to get in touch with the donor brother. It was just an anxious waiting time for us doctors and the family.

One cannot even imagine what happened next. The clock kept ticking as our anxiety mounted.

Three hours later – around mid-day – we got to know that a young man was admitted with head injury in the casualty department of Safdarjung Hospital, across the road and a packet of some injections addressed to AIIMS were in his bag.

The Delhi Transport Corporation bus, which was plying from Palam airport into the city, had stopped on the left side of the road, facing north, and a young man getting off the footboard had a serious fall. People on the pavement and the police had rushed him to the hospital nearest. And this is how, he was admitted in Safdarjung hospital and not in All India Institute – a thin line in the middle of this road divides the police jurisdiction between these two hospitals even today.

As soon as we got the information, we realised, the accident victim was connected to our transplant case waiting to get on the table.

I remember, as the principal nephrologist in charge of the case, I rushed to the casualty department of Safdarjung hospital only to discover that the young man who was lying unconscious in the casualty was our donor. Time was of prime importance to us, but no ambulance was available at that moment to just take one patient across the road to AIIMS from the Safdarjung hospital.

Under my signature, my staff and I transported the young man on a trolley, pushing it across the road.

The different police personnel – ours and theirs, jurisdiction-wise – were asked to wait. The accident victim was put on the ventilator and given all necessary treatment. He remained alive for a day and passed away on the very day of the scheduled kidney transplantation.

It was the most tragic episode to date for all of us at AIIMS. The family was distraught. So were we. And in those days, at the beginning of the nephrological services in the country, our hospital departments were not smart enough to perform cadaver transfer at once. Neither were the family nor were the hospitals mentally ready, and it was a tragic and emotional moment for all of us.

We lost two perfectly usable healthy kidneys on that day – we had not planned for any such contingency and the human element that is always at play in these cases. In those days, harvesting an organ from the dead was considered sacrilege and even to suggest it to a bereaved family would have been unthinkable, even at AIIMS. We did not do the planned transplant on the brother with end-stage kidney failure and in the end failed to save this brother too.

The loss of a life, however, was not the end of this unfortunate episode. We learnt soon that the young wife of the prospective donor brother had committed suicide by hanging from a ceiling fan at home, while all other members were in the hospital dealing with the unfortunate death.

It was a situation one cannot comprehend. A situation where two lives – that of the prospective donor and his wife – were lost in total futility.

I hate to write this – we did not have a practice of cadaver (dead body) organ removal during that period and two human lives, four perfectly good kidneys, were lost in such a hurricane short period of 24 hours, amidst acute shortage of kidneys for transplant. At least four people could have been given a boon of life from these two young cadavers, including the needy brother.

This very painful incident still haunts me even after fifty-five years in the profession, no matter how hard I try not to think of this family that lost three lives in quick succession.

I sit down to pen my thoughts today, with the people of India in mind, who knowingly or unknowingly are a part of this huge racket I talk about in a kidney trade, flourishing illegally only in India. No other country in the world – with much poorer and less educated people – is home to a nation-wide scam that is taking place in India, despite stringent laws.

Tardy enforcement and human greed are not the only factors promoting illegal kidney donations. It is lack of ethics in the individual, big and small, rich and poor, doctor and patient, the scamster and law keeping agencies, the legislators and courts which has made India a bazaar for kidneys, harvested illegally, with forged papers. And one must remember,

A WORD FROM MY HEART

it is only India's poor who are duped into selling their kidney, India's rich are as much recipients of purchased kidneys as anyone else in the rest of the world. In this country of one billion plus people, bring me one 'poor' recipient of nephrological services and a kidney donated. There are no religious overtones or cultural compulsions here except the 'rich and poor' divide. I write with sadness in my heart and a bleak vision of the future of my people, considered 'purchasable' by the rest of the world.

PREFACE

The latter half of the 20th century saw immense progress in India in the field of nephrology – the branch of medicine which addresses the diseases of kidney function.

The first successful renal transplant in India took place in 1971 at the Christian Medical College, Vellore, and an exclusive department for kidney diseases was set up in the All India Institute of Medical Sciences, New Delhi in 1972. However, as nephrology flourished in the seventies, a large percentage of kidney donors insidiously changed from relatives of the recipients to unrelated groups.

Amidst blatant commercialism, there was open soliciting in print media by the families of patients or unscrupulous individuals who appeared on behalf of the recipients with cash offers. This is how a clean practice of kidney transplantation got vitiated in the country. At the time, there were no guidelines or checks by health authorities, and as the abundance of transplant centres increased, so did the availability of 'distant cousins' who arrived as apparent living related donors. The brokers and middlemen became central to the enterprise. With no legislation in place, there was little agreement in the medical community about the ethics of organ purchase and putting an end to live, unrelated kidney donation.

It was in the eighties that India became the 'Kidney Bazaar' of the world, where foreigners arrived as medical tourists to purchase organs from the non-literate and impoverished class. Initially, Mumbai was the epicentre of the 'Kidney Trade' because of its proximity to the Gulf and African countries. This practice quickly spread to Madras (Chennai), Calcutta (Kolkata), Bangalore (Bengaluru) and ultimately reached the north in places like Delhi and Punjab, devouring prominent hospitals in the wake of its tragedy.

The Government of India passed The Transplantation of Human Organs Act in 1994, modified it in 2011 and in 2014 to The Transplantation of Human Organs and Tissues Act. Neither THOA 1994 nor the THOTA of 2014 have been able to put a stop to this clandestine, exploitative, inhumane and illegal trade so openly practiced in the country.

In 2008, in Moradabad, Uttar Pradesh, local police combined with the efforts of Delhi and Haryana Police teams, raided a hospital run illegally by the kingpin of one of the largest kidney scams in the country: There were five donors who had been operated upon and their kidneys harvested and their lives were in danger as they were, theoretically, still in-patients. They all had undergone kidney donating operations on the day the hospital was raided. Suddenly they were told, just a few minutes before police came in, that 'the doctor has been caught and the police is coming'. So, what did the hospital staff do? They removed all the blood drips and glucose tubes from these donors on the various beds and said, 'You also run away from here'.

Their kidneys were harvested just a few hours earlier, and they were dangerously shooed away from the so-called hospital and abandoned and there was no one to take care of them. Media reports at the time said, 'one of the patients was actually writhing in pain'.

In another gruesome incident, the victim was a young woman in Kolkata who, after her marriage in 2005, remained under constant pressure to bring dowry for her husband and his family. In India, dowry, again, is a social bane, which cannot be controlled despite laws against the practice.

In 2016, this young woman was admitted to a hospital for an appendectomy and her kidney was illegally harvested. The police arrested the woman's husband and his brother from Murshidabad district near Kolkata. The husband then confessed that he had sold her kidney to a businessman in Chhattisgarh. This particular case had attracted the attention of foreign media, including the *Telegraph* and the *Washington Post*.

Such episodes of scams and exploitation of the poor have continued till the time of writing this book and I cannot pronounce in words that there will be a complete halt to this crime in my lifetime.

MY BLACKENED FACE

Doctors are often accused of callousness and self-infatuation – believed to be people who exploit fellow humans in pain and with health problems. On the other hand, in India, they are placed at par or next to God. In this process, the Doctor oscillates like a pendulum at his work and becomes a tool in the hands of his patients and their families and others in society.

India is a developing country, economically. The nation's assets are shared unequally by 133.92 crore people or nearly 1.4 billion people. According to the latest government data: India's gross domestic product is estimated to have slowed to a five-year low of 5.8 per cent in the last quarter of fiscal ended March 2018–2019. At the same time, the country's per capita income is estimated to have risen by 10 per cent to ₹10,534 a month during the financial year ended March 2019, government data on national income showed in June. In 2017–2018, the monthly per-capita income had stood at ₹9,580. This does not mean every adult Indian has ₹10,000 to spend every month even as Chandrayan 3 gets ready for another moon mission.

In the last fifty years, since the 1970s, India has progressed rapidly in healthcare indices, yet the anomalies are stupefying. The Maternal Mortality Rate has declined from 167 in 2011–2013 to 130 in 2014–2016 per 100,000 live births, according to a special health bulletin from the government in 2018. Still, about 44 children out of 1,000 live births die even today. Yet, India has emerged as one of the top 10 medical tourism destinations in the world with more than four lakh people visiting India annually for low-cost healthcare that range from heart transplant to knee surgery and Ayurveda, amounting to about 5 per cent of the total yearly tourism revenue – about ₹200,000 crore. And India is also where kidneys can be bought for a few lakh of rupees. The poor in India, however, have no access to even basic healthcare, and certainly no access to dialysis or kidney transplants even in major government-run hospitals. What is low-cost for the world is unaffordable to the poor Indian.

The majority of people in India are Hindus. Poverty, among Hindus, is said to be a result of *karma* – deeds done in earlier lives as well as in the current life – where even the current life is a result of pervious *karma*, good or bad. The 'poor' in India is deprived, uneducated and always in need of funds. S/he remains at the end of the economic supply chain, which includes basic housing, schooling and medicare and often gets nothing in her/his life. Doctors fall in the high-income bracket, at the high end of the economic supply chain by virtue of being educated. This, however, does not decrease their 'irresistible desire' for more, nor does their swearing by the Hippocratic Oath make them any more ethical than the average medically untrained human being. The healer and the poor are all caught in the web of a nation-wide trade in kidneys perpetuated by rich recipients, their families and middlemen – all five categories of people making up the innards of a runaway scam that no government in India is able to reign in.

The authorities, as well as civil society, acknowledge that the 'kidney rackets' need a final solution. After all, who is responsible for such ongoing rackets all over India, in almost every big and small city? A solution is necessary for the exploited poor and also for the acclaimed and senior kidney physicians in the country, accused of unethical organ harvesting or being part of bad hospital management or just watching silently without contributing to stemming the rot in the system.

As a specialist nephrologist, I have participated in the emergence of the much-needed kidney transplantation service in major hospitals in the country from its beginning in the early seventies to the present time and I have witnessed the various forces at work in this field of healthcare. In the '80s and '90s, our country was labeled as the 'Kidney Bazaar' of the world. But subsequently, with the enactment of The Transplantation of Human Organs Act, 1994 (THOA), this image and the practice of ethical kidney transplantation did improve immensely. This is, however, a case of too little, too late.

Even today, two decades into the 21st century, the fact remains that we keep hearing of such painful incidents from time to time. With technological advances, kidney scandals, scams and the trade of kidneys has gone out of hand of governments, hospitals and civil society.

Are the various doctors engaged in transplantation squarely responsible for these malpractices?

My answer is – No!

The treatment and activity of kidney transplantation is done by well-trained, fairly well-to-do and senior persons in their profession. I cannot accept that one of us would participate in a racket, put his/her life's reputation in the hands of others and then languish in jail.

The fact is that a kidney physician/surgeon remains totally vulnerable to the suffering, hardship and pressures of his patient who wishes to survive at any cost. That is where the whole story begins. The catchword is: *Survive at any cost.* Irrespective of what happens to anyone else. Irrespective of the right and wrong of it.

Doctors are often inadvertently pushed into the process of these duplicity/rackets happening in India. High-profile patients like 'NRIs, businessmen, politicians and bureaucrats' pressure the treating doctor, the specialist.

India's laws don't help much either. The doctor/surgeon is an expert in performing the kidney replacement operation. *S/he is NOT an expert in documentation and verification.* This operating specialist is most often made to speak to unknown donors and their agents – presented to him as 'friends or relatives (cousins)' by the family of the prospective recipient. The doctors cannot distinguish/detect the impersonation, fictitious albeit genuine-looking relatives, and the relevant documents presented to the hospital or the State Authorisation Committees for approval. One specialist has many patients in any hospital or private clinic settings. The doctor knows how to give medical care. *S/he does not know if a piece of paper or a certificate is genuine or not. If a family, donor, recipient is telling the truth or lies.*

Fabricating fake documents is a huge industry in itself; this is a malady of high magnitude and nearly insurmountable at this stage. Hospitals do not have lie detectors or security-police scanners that can detect fake documents and lies. Nor do average authorisation committees have psychiatrists on panels, though this is legally mandatory. In an attempt to plug the loopholes, the Transplantation Act has been modified twice – in 2011 and 2014. However, ambiguities in the law continue to remain.

The present law permits transplantation from totally 'unrelated donor' source – after it is verified and authenticated by the duly-appointed 'hospital-based Authorisation Committee', of which the treating doctor is not a member.

Any member of this 'authorisation committee' can be open to 'pressure' from political quarters, the rich and the famous, a peer group or hospital bosses. Any member of such a 'authorisation committee' can just as well knowingly connive to okay fake documents and transplants based on these. Any member of such a 'authorisation committee' can be also too trusting of his/her assisting staff and hospital facilitators and managers and can be duped. The blame rarely reaches the 'authorisation committee' members and hospital managers and auxiliary staff.

Mostly, it is the care-taking doctor and operating surgeon who are named, hauled up, humiliated and his/her character assassinated.

For this doctor/surgeon, often, the reality is that there is a 'donor' on the table and a 'recipient' on the second table who have both arrived at the operation theatre through the hospital system. He is not likely to guess that the donor–recipient are not related. Or that the documentation of the donor is false. Even if they are not related, the matching of blood and tissue and the compatibility test is verified by the 'authorisation committee', supposed to be designated by the hospital and experts in their field. Look at the catch in the situation. The recipient is real. The donor is real. Only the papers of the donor are fudged.

Thus, the doctor who was next to God one moment, has his 'face blackened' without any means of protesting or proving himself/herself innocent. S/he has committed the crime of harvesting a kidney from a donor who has 'sold' it to the recipient. Quite often, these days, the doctor does everything in good faith but becomes a victim of his own doings. He remains under police surveillance as a 'criminal' and is bundled into a lockup without being allowed a whimper! What an irony!

The culprits are those groups of undesirable characters who exploit any situation of 'demand' and enter into money transaction to 'supply' that demand – a kind of prostitution in organ trade.

The real culprits – the middlemen, touts, hospital staff involved and various others who have participated knowingly – put the medical profession in the dark.

In India, not only kidneys but heart, liver and skin are sold as well. A patient with low blood platelet count has accused a doctor at a specialty hospital of advising her to get her spleen removed!

Whenever a case or scam comes under media glare, the police in various medical centres reap a rich harvest too. They get paid by the recipient family not to pursue investigation and not to file charges; they make money from the arrested to 'complicate' the case, to mishandle 'evidence'; they make money to let arrested culprits escape; they get publicity, promotions and ensure that the case proceeds in the court/s for unlimited period of time, without any conviction and punishment. The humiliated doctor, his family and the cheated slum dwellers continue to suffer throughout their lives.

One is often forced to wonder why does the press wake up only when something sensational happens? Why cannot the media keep a continuous eye on the kidney/organ commerce in the country?

The solution to this malady is in identifying the middleman who is the 'actual kingpin' warranting severe punishment. The relatives of kidney patients and the conniving hospital staff should also be punished. The so-called 'cousins' of a patient – the kidney-selling donor – and kidney-buying recipient should also be brought under the purview of law with equal punishment. And these punishments should include a huge economic component because it is money that is driving the kidney trade today.

Our country tops in the world in road traffic accidents and in Delhi and the National Capital Region alone, about 6 to 7 people meet fatal accidents daily. *Harvesting of kidneys from unfortunate accident victims is the only solution to the shortage of kidneys for transplantation in India.*

We all need to urgently respond to this task both at the government level and with amendment of available laws to remove organs from brain-dead victims, with consent of the families. It is a gigantic task. The awareness of organ donation from cadaveric source is of paramount importance in this country.

My slogan has been and continues to be ONE LIFE SAVES FOUR LIVES. Two available kidneys save two persons' lives and in turn they also vacate life-saving dialysis machines for two other patients. *I do not want to see this final solution remain just a dream in my lifetime!*

INTRODUCTION

A live kidney weighing 150–200gms is the most sought-after organ worldwide and there is a ready market of people willing to sell for an attractive price.

THE KIDNEYS ARE A PAIR of organs present in between the vertebrates of human beings. They receive blood from the renal arteries, separate the urine from the blood and expel the cleaner blood from the renal veins; each kidney is connected to a ureter which carries excreted urine to the bladder. The kidneys serve to control the volume of various body fluids in various compartments of the body, fluid osmolality, acid-base balance in the body, various electrolyte concentrations, and they help remove toxins (poisonous substances) from the body.

In ancient Indian literature, the presence of sugar in urine was described during 3000–4000 BC. People had found that they could use ants to test for a sugar-related condition of the body by presenting urine to them. If the ants came to the urine, this was a sign that it contained high sugar levels. They called the condition *madhumeha*, meaning honey urine. This is described in detail in texts like *Charaka* and *Sushruta,* the *Samihta*s dated to about 300 years BC. At that time urine was specifically connected to the body organ, kidneys. The Greek historian Diodorus Siculus (between 90 BC – 30 BC in Italy) wrote that Egyptian embalmers did not extract the kidneys, along with the heart, prior to mummification, considering the organs to be 'unimportant' and difficult to excise.

KIDNEY DISEASES AND TREATMENT MODALITIES

All mammals have two kidneys and in outlier cases a single kidney may be present. Though both kidneys work simultaneously, if one becomes dysfunctional or is removed for transplantation in another individual, a single kidney works fairly well during a normal lifespan.

Inflammation of the tiny filters in the kidneys (glomeruli) is called glomerulo-nephritis. Glomeruli remove excess fluid, electrolytes and waste from our bloodstream and pass them into our urine.

Diabetes mellitus is a metabolic disease that causes high blood sugar. The hormone insulin moves sugar from the blood into our cells to be stored or used for energy. With diabetes, our body either doesn't make enough insulin or can't effectively use the insulin it does make. Untreated high blood sugar from diabetes can damage our nerves, eyes, kidneys and other organs.

Similarly, long-standing and poorly controlled hypertension damages kidney structure and causes failure. Other diseases too affect kidneys and cause damage to kidneys in similar ways – not to forget familial diseases like polycystic kidneys and congenital malformation. There is now an uncontrollable contributory factor of high analgesic (pain killers) usage in middle-aged persons, leading to chronic kidney failure.

Kidney diseases have many causes, while kidney failure is predominantly of two different types:

Acute Kidney Injury (AKI) – wherein the kidneys acutely stop functioning, which is also called acute kidney failure. With AKI, there is a possibility of reversing the damage with treatment in a hospital setup. In some cases, fluid and electrolyte replacement is required and most cases have complicating infections. Treatment includes the institution of hemodialysis support. AKI can occur at any age.

Chronic Kidney Disease (CKD) – is an incurable disease caused by multiple factors. It occurs primarily after the age of 30 years and has a progressive course.

There is little reliable data available in India and other developing countries about the occurrence of CKD. However, there is rise in its occurrence in these countries. China and India, the two most populous nations, and countries such as Pakistan and Indonesia also witness high incidence of CKD.

In India, rough estimates indicate that 100,000 to 130,000 new CKD patients seek treatment in a year, not including patients in rural areas who do not receive medical attention at all.

THE WHY OF IT

The top three factors causing CKD in India are diabetes mellitus, hypertension and chronic glomerulonephritis. Diseases like kidney stones, neglected kidney infections, obstructive uropathy (a condition when urine cannot drain through the urinary tract. Urine backs up into the kidney and causes it to become swollen) and gout also contribute to the development of CKD.

Amyloid are a number of complex proteins that are deposited in tissues and that share selected laboratory features such as a change in the fluorescence intensity of certain aromatic dyes like Congo Red. The deposition of amyloid occurs in a number of diseases. In many of these, there is disagreement as to whether amyloid causes the disease or is simply a sign of the disease.

Diseases that cause the deposition of amyloids in kidneys, tuberculosis, excessive use of analgesics (over-the-counter painkillers) and auto-immune disorders involving kidneys also add to the development of CKD.

Chronic Kidney Disease (CKD stage 5), also known as End Stage Renal Disease (ESRD) – is a multi-factorial and diabetic chronic kidney disease. This is most prevalent among Indian populations, accounting for as much as 45–50 per cent of the patients coming into hospitals for treatment. Its frequency is reported to be rising at an alarming pace in South Asia.

Diabetic kidney in younger patients in India is also seen with alarming rapidity.

The World Health Organisation predicts a 170–200% increase in Type 2 Diabetes with 90–100 million diabetic people in India alone with every

4th diabetic of the world an Indian by 2025. The co-morbid conditions are increasing proportionally. (Co-morbid is a common medical term. 'Comorbidity' refers to one or more diseases or conditions that occur along with another condition in the same person at the same time. Conditions considered comorbid are often long-term or chronic conditions.)

Evidence suggests that very rapid urbanisation, industrialisation and technological advancement all lead to physical inactivity and obesity, which contribute to Type 2 diabetes in the younger population of India. Sometimes, diabetes is genetically inherited. However, there is no accurate and broad-based National or Regional reports/registry on incidence or prevalence of either CKD or end-stage renal disease (ESRD) in the country yet. This enumeration is still at a preliminary stage.

ESRD, in its relentless course, carries multiple co-morbid conditions such as hypertension, cardio-vascular disease, cerebro-vascular disease, dyslipidemia, crippling neuropathies, worsening vision and malnutrition.

The current extensive research in different areas of diabetic nephropathies for genetic basis, linkage of high blood sugar levels with hypertension, structural kidney damage, improvement in protein loss and kidney function impairment has been encouraging but inconclusive.

Hypertension is labeled as a silent killer and affects all major organs like the brain, heart, kidneys, eyes, and major blood vessels of human body. The incidence of hypertension is much higher in males than females. In recent years, younger people in their twenties and thirties have been affected. The importance of effective and regular treatment of hypertension is poorly understood and compliance is totally inadequate.

In India, a vast country of 1.3 billion people, early identification is lacking, and hypertension is detected only when a serious complication like stroke, cardiac disease or chronic kidney disease has set in.

Excessive usage of painkillers is a worldwide problem and its importance in progression in CKD is poorly recognised. Over-the-counter availability and low cost lead to widespread consumption and an individual has very little insight of complications with drugs called NSAIDs (non-steroidal anti-inflammatory drugs). Its usage by elderly patients of osteoarthritis, spondylitis, headaches and even tiredness is common. These drugs contribute to the progressive decline of kidneys.[1]

Indigenous Medicines: In India and China, indigenous drugs are used frequently, and these countries remain a hub of supply.

The ancient teachings of Ayurveda and traditional Chinese medicines have their place in certain selected diseases at present times. The claims of 'effective cure of diabetes mellitus', hypertension or chronic kidney disease are unsubstantiated by clinically recorded evidence and their regular use appears to more often than not complicate and worsen the progression of CKD.

[1] https://bmcnephrol.biomedcentral.com/articles/10.1186/1471-2369-13-10

Ironically, public education on these products in print and visual media is rampant and these drugs are available online and easily procured even at licensed chemist shops. The state encouragement for the development of indigenous medicine has pitfalls in chronic diseases and in surgical conditions. However – that many patients turn to explore the avenue of alternative medicine – is understandable.

The Wonder of Science: There have been multiple wonders and enormous strides in the field of medical science in the last fifty years. Medical technology has advanced in every sphere of human care including stem cell therapy, regeneration of human cells, genetic modification of hereditary disease i.e. polycystic kidneys, Huntington's chorea and there are even attempts to generate human organs in sight.

Since Chronic Kidney Disease is irreversible, patients have no choice and require Renal Replacement Therapy (RRT). During the course of the illness too, the patient is burdened with endless problems. The prospect of a long-term treatment plan is devastating to the patient and painful and trying for their family. In most cases, such a treatment plan remains unmanageable and incomplete. This picture is largely uniform in India and other developing countries.

The creation of artificial kidney (dialysis) in sustaining human life is the most spectacular among developments available to the common man. The procedures of dialysis include hemodialysis, peritoneal dialysis and continuous ambulatory peritoneal dialysis (CAPD).

In India: Currently, hemodialysis is widely accepted across the world. Such centres are confined to the cities in India, while 65 per cent of our population still live in rural areas. Those seeking hemodialysis treatment are just about 10% of all patients to begin with. The rate of those who opt out of such treatment (the drop rate) for various reasons appears to be 95%.

For this small group of patients seeking long-term hemodialysis, state-funded and insurance-supported schemes are a miniscule alternative for a shorter period.

India is a heterogeneous country where health-related schemes are a State subject; national health schemes sponsored by the central government are insufficient to provide comprehensive coverage to the entire population of the country. Since government institutions are unable to provide full care, optimum benefit and outcome of maintenance, the hemodialysis programme remains unsatisfactory throughout the country. At the government-level India is a poor service provider. As such, the talk of India being or even becoming a 'developed country' or 'an advanced medicare tourism destination' is just so much talk.

With this dismal condition of State-funded health care programmes, patients go to multiple hospitals to seek treatment for various ailments at their own expenses. Private hospitals remain an overly expensive proposition for most patients.

In India, the hemodialysis machines and disposable kidneys are exclusively imported, even after four decades of starting such facilities. We might be building satellites and our own pins, buckets and cars, and have a national strategy for artificial intelligence (AI), or our IT sector may earn us revenues of US$160 billion (in 2017 according to NASSCOM) but India has yet to come up with affordable dialysis machines.[2]

Dialysis machines are now imported from Germany, Sweden and China (yes even China) at a cost of ₹10–11 lakh a unit. This makes the cost of one session of dialysis between ₹3,000–5,000. Though India has made a nascent beginning, wide reach and affordability of India-made machines will take some decades to become a reality for the common man.

The Financial Burden: As of now, high margins levied by private hospitals keep the dialysis cost high and provide poor dialysis support without any quality control or proper management, and most

---

[2] Designed by Renalyx Health Systems, the first made-in-India machine, RxT17, started undergoing trials at the JSS Medical College Hospital in the southern city of Mysore in March 2018. The first patient was a 40-year-old man.

The machine is cloud-enabled and can be connected to a mobile app for nephrologists to be able to monitor its functioning. Also, the patient response.

Shyam Vasudev Rao, an Indian Institute of Science (IISc) alumnus and founder scientist of Renalyx Health Systems says, the machine can be taken to rural areas, and operates on solar power too. Not even Japanese and US machines have such enabling features.

Dr Lloyd Vincent, a nephrologist and co-founder of Renalyx, says the production must be cost-effective. 'The object is to reduce costs.'

'We have a project monitoring committee with alumni from Bombay and Delhi IITs as well as AIIMS. The project has been funded by the Department of Science and Technology, Government of India.'

http://timesofindia.indiatimes.com/articleshow/63250621.cms?utm_source=contentofinterest&utm_medium=text&utm_campaign=cppst

patients are able to afford hemodialysis for only a short period.

With financial constraints and overwhelming pressure, patients then choose hemodialysis for infrequent intervals voluntarily. With initial improvement in health – all constraints appear of lesser consequence, although the quality of life is affected significantly.

The economics of any type of RRT is enormous and becomes a final point in the determination of treatment of CKD in most cases in India and less-economically developed countries across the world.

Financial constraints become the foremost consideration in most cases. In the absence of state-sponsored financial support systems available to all, the meager help from insurance or employers remains insufficient and the burden falls on the patient. While accepting any treatment modality on a long-term basis, the quality of life and cost of living become a prime consideration for most people. For patients, normal life is changed to just a process of prolonging life for the person – and spouse, parents and others suffer enormously.

This is a major factor in the well-being of a person with CKD which urgently needs attention and requires professional management advisory.

CURES AND COSTS

THE TRUTH OF THE MATTER is, a bad kidney is a bad kidney. It is like a bad eye.

To modify vision of a defective eye, one can wear a spectacle. That is a management decision, to go to an eye doctor, get your vision checked, wear powered glasses, use medicine drops or have a cataract operation or surgically rectify vision any other way, or in extreme cases, have an eye donation and transplant. Similarly, for a kidney.

A bad kidney has to be managed.

One can go to a doctor, go to a specialist, take medicines like diuretics, then depending on need and condition, go on dialysis. Ultimately, when all else fails, like one can wear someone else's eye – one can wear someone else's kidney.

This is a theoretical proposition. Even in India, no one is gouging out anyone else's eyes. There are two eyes. One can see perfectly well with one eye. So, why don't poor people sell one of their eyes? Why kidney?

This can be a matter of general perception and belief. In many cultures, the eye is considered a jewel – a window to the mind. Eyes are associated with beauty. Eye can be seen by the viewer opposite. Eye can be beautiful or scary or terrified – it is an external expression of 'expression'. Not even the poorest of the poor 'sell' an eye. Yet, eye operations and transplants are routine in India. Cadaver organ harvesting for the eyes is now a general practice, donating eyes by terminally ill patients serve more than an altruistic purpose.

Kidney, on the other hand, is associated with a process of excretion – it is invisible, hidden somewhere deep inside the body. It is mentally associated with something 'unclean' in the Indian psyche. This is one reason, often even relatives with matching blood groups refuse to donate kidneys. That someone else's body waste will be filtered through 'my kidney' is not a happy idea. So rich families opt to buy kidneys from the unrelated poor though a relative donor may be available. The semi-literate poor do not know the inner anatomy of a human body. The hands are to eat with, legs to walk with, if you close your eyes, you cannot see, so eyes are to see with. Rest of the body is a mystery to him or her.

When a semi-literate poor is shown a picture of inner body organs – s/he is shown one heart and large liver lobes and told there are two lungs (which cannot be harvested as it helps one to breath – again an external factor s/he can identified with at once) and two kidneys, both excreting – the prospective donor associates the kidney with *dispensability*.

'Performs an excretory function, have two – one works just as well' – an understanding that is flawed and fueled by the prospect also of monetisation.

So, the first issue for India is to make the common man understand body parts and their basic functions. This may help change the mindset somewhat. It may need a huge awareness campaign to make the ordinary individual understand that any 'organ' is *not* dispensable or throw-away, every organ in the body has a purpose and is precious. There are two lungs and two kidneys for a reason. To stop the current manner of trading in kidneys, to steer a mindset change would need a national campaign. Logic has to supersede fear and greed.

It is only then that any treatment for kidney-related illnesses can be completely managed. Be it within a home system or a hospital system.

The next important step would perhaps be to bridge the patient-specialist gap, given that there are less than 1,500 nephrologists in India for her 1.3 billion people.

THE AVAILABLE OPTIONS

Hemodialysis (blood dialysis): This is performed in hospitals and dialysis centres. In India, the concept of 'home dialysis' is rare and has been only possible for a high-profile patient like the former Prime Minister of India, Vishwanath Pratap Singh.

This procedure is performed three times in a week, but many patients accept it twice in a week. Because of the cost and because of less availability of the dialysis machines – two factors that play primary roles in treatment management.

Each procedure is for four hours and sometimes requires special monitoring i.e. oxygen and cardiac monitoring, and blood transfusion when necessary.

In most dialysis units there is a 'dialyser re-use system' from two to eight sittings to minimise the cost for the patient and for gain by hospitals. Hemodialyser reuse refers to the practice of using the same dialyser (artificial blood-urine interphase membrane) multiple times for a single patient. Reuse was commonly practiced in the United States during the 1980s through 1990s, and it was believed that as much as 40 per cent patients were on reuse mode. This was for cost containment but also to reduce the incidence of inflammatory reactions due to blood-membrane interactions with bio-incompatible cellulose membranes. Today, in the USA, reuse of dialyser has reduced but 'reuse' is still commonly done in other parts of the world. Only hollow fiber dialysers that are labeled by the manufacturer for multiple use are reprocessed and reused thus.[1]

The charges of hemodialysis vary widely, and patients often have to choose the nearest and cheapest option, with no regard to quality of hemodialysis, and hospitals and institutions offering dialysis are always at a greater advantage of earnings on the whole.

The use of erythropoietin, parenteral vitamin supplements and drugs used for muscle cramps add to the cost.

---

[1] https://www.uptodate.com/contents/reuse-of-dialyzers

The regular schedule of hemodialysis is not adhered to by all patients which can lead to fluid overload, respiratory, cardiac distress and other emergencies. Anemia is seen in practically all patients due to multiple factors of disease, poor iron intake, recurrent blood loss and inability to respond to erythropoietin therapy. It causes fatigue and constitutional morbidities. Folic acid, vitamin-B12 and parenteral iron are needed on a regular basis and these most patients cannot afford on a long-term.

Diet and water restrictions are extremely binding – and following these two constraints are most important to the maintenance of hemodialysis. Any deviation in water intake leads to worsening of hypertension, heart failure, respiratory problems and fluid retention, leading to other serious medical complications.

The poor nutrition, self-restriction of protein intake, pre-dominant vegetarian diet with absent essential amino-acids causes protein negative balance, progressive weight loss and malnutrition resulting in poor health with constant fatigue and increased susceptibility to infections.

The problems of anorexia and ill health are compounded by depression. Other limitations such as insufficient physical activity and sleep disorders are frequently seen. The problems of sexual dysfunction and significant alteration of menstrual cycle are also common. The components of depression and diabetes mellitus compound decreased libido.

The invisible expenses of transportation, medicines, and investigations lead to further strain on the patient's mental and physical health.

The problem of pain becomes of musculoskeletal-type due to poor nutrition, renal bone disease, absence of physical exercise and in some patients, it is even psychosomatic in nature.

There are frequent episodes of infection related to internal jugular and femoral catheters (passages/tubes) used for longer periods of hemodialysis maintenance. These catheter-related infections are compounded by the funding restrictions in Employees State Insurance Scheme (ESIC in India) and Ex-servicemen Contributory Health Scheme (ECHS in India) rules and regulations, resulting in delays in required treatment.[2]

Other infections such as respiratory, urinary or systemic are also seen frequently in chronic kidney disease patients. Water treatment plants (i.e. RO or Kent system) are only installed in major hospitals as plants are expensive and most centres compromise on the quality of water used. The surveillance of bacterial contamination is not rigid, endotoxins, episodes of shivering, high fever and use of expensive antibiotics result in longer periods of hospitalisation.

Life-long hemodialysis treatment may also lead to failure of vascular access, loss of energy and ability to work. Age becomes a major factor in the well-being of a person, and as normal routine is changed to

---

[2] As I elaborate in Appendix C, ESIC funding do not necessarily support kidney transplant. –Author

prolong life, this, unfortunately, has to be accepted under all circumstances. Upon any improvement in the multiple symptoms, the feeling of relief of 'a life saved' is soon complicated by treatment restrictions, burden of institutional treatment, financial constraints and changes in employment.

Chronic Ambulatory Peritoneal Dialysis (CAPD): This was introduced to India by the author (Dr Ramesh Kumar) while working at AIIMS forty-five years ago with a grant given by the Indian Council of Medical Research (ICMR) in 1973–74.

This procedure is provided to elderly patients over the age of 65 years, patients with poor cardiac function, limitation of vascular access and some patients who do not want maintenance hemodialysis or kidney transplantation.

This procedure is done with placement of a special catheter (Tenckhoff) in the lower abdomen and commercially available fluid for CAPD is instilled thrice a day either manually or with a cycler machine.

The patient's own peritoneal membrane (covering on intestinal loops) serves as a filtration membrane for all components of the dialysis procedure. The acceptance of CAPD is easier as regular treatment is done at home. The monthly cost is comparable to institutionally maintained hemodialysis and long-term outcome for selected patient is better in terms of improvement of health and longevity.

The limitations of CAPD include daily treatment, infection and exhaustion of the permeability of the peritoneal membrane. On the other hand, dietary and water restrictions get eliminated and the patient feels in command of his treatment. The diabetes control requires high doses of insulin.

Overall, it is a readily accepted treatment modality by the spouse and immediate family who can afford the cost or expenses are state-sponsored. The young working patients are not offered CAPD and nephrologists generally recommend kidney transplantation, which is most suitable for them.

Kidney Transplantation: In developing countries, a desirable and widely-accepted modality of RRT is a kidney transplant.

It is a one-time surgical procedure, and the regular follow-ups are undertaken at increasing intervals. The recipient is required to take life-long immnosuppressive medication, with the exception of a few instances of identical twins. In early periods, incidence of complications with infection and bone marrow suppression were seen more frequently. With the advent of better drugs, kidney transplantation appears to be a well-established mode of treatment of CKD. The surgical techniques have improved significantly, and transplants are done in all major cities across the country.

In India, a majority of the legal kidney transplantation is from living, related donors and peri-operative death rate ranges from less than 1% for donors and less than 5% for recipient.

Laparoscopic nephrectomy (separating the donor kidney) has now become the preferred surgical procedure and is increasingly practiced. The graft survival is 98% at Year One and there is a 5% deduction to this success on a yearly basis.

Human Leukocyte Antigen (HLA)[3] matching is done uniformly in all transplant centres and has greatly contributed to the success of kidney transplantation. This ensures that the immune system of the recipient does not violently oppose the donated kidney as the recipent's HLA is similar to the donor's.

The limitations of kidney transplantation include regular intake of immunosuppressive agents, opportunistic infections, development of post-operative diabetes, hypertension and the burden of regular follow-up. Nevertheless, for both, the doctor and the patient, transplantation remains a prioritised and satisfying modality of RRT.

In a majority of cases, one kidney from the donor is transplanted into the recipient. In the last five years, among two unrelated couples in a 'swap category', kidneys have been transplanted to the most suitable recipient from the four people involved.

Kidney transplantation is now even practiced from pediatric age groups to patients in their seventies with CKD.

The major surgical steps undertaken are that the donor renal artery is connected to the external iliac artery of the recipient. And the donor renal vein is connected to external iliac vein in the recipient. The ureter of donor is anastomosed[4] through a

---

[3] The human leukocyte antigen (HLA) system or complex is a gene system encoding the major histocompatibility complex (MHC) proteins in humans. These cell-surface proteins are responsible for the regulation of the immune system in humans.

[4] An anastomosis is a connection or opening between two things (especially cavities or passages) that are normally diverging or branching, such as between blood vessels, leaf veins, or streams.

tunnel made in the recipient's bladder. *The diseased kidneys of the recipient are not removed except under specific conditions* before transplantation.

Thus, a recipient carries three kidneys of which only the transplanted kidney is functioning to sustain normal health. In certain cases, a dual kidney – pancreas transplant is undertaken in diabetic patients. The transplant surgery is performed in 3–5 hours and urine flow is immediate on the operating table. The kidney function returns to normal range between 3–5 days.

The donor is discharged in less than 7 days and the recipient requires 8–10 days of hospital stay. The laparoscopic removal of kidney from donor entails a shorter hospital stay.

The common immunosuppressive drugs to suppress the immune system of recipient so that it does not reject the donated kidney are prednisolone, tacrolimus and mycophenolate mofetil.

A serial set of investigations is done on a daily basis. Monitoring of tacrolimus level (the level of an immunosupressant agent) in blood is done periodically until the level is stabilised between 10–15ng/ml.[5]

Major complications of transplantation include rejection of the donated kidney by the recipient immune system. These rejections are classified as hyper acute (within hours), acute or acute in chronic stage – in later stages of transplantation. Other

---

Such a connection may be normal or abnormal, naturally occurring or done by a surgical intervention.

[5] https://www.ncbi.nlm.nih.gov/pubmed/22128417

problems that may occur are infections, fluid and electrolyte imbalances, worsening of hypertension, urinary protein loss and side effects of immuno-suppressive agents.

The lifespan of a kidney transplant varies from 10–15 years and can be improved upon with meticulous post-transplant care. In the experience of this author, a set of five transplant patients are living for more than 35 years, with their donor kidneys. This is, however, a rare case.

Cadaver Kidney Transplantation: This was made possible in India with the passing of the Transplantation of Human Organs Act (THOA) in 1994. In this procedure, a kidney is removed from a brain-dead individual with a beating heart.

There are well-prescribed procedural guidelines given under the notification of the National Organ and Tissue Transplant Organisation (NOTTO). The prospective donor remains on life support systems (for example, a ventilator) and his life span varies from 15–20 years. A prospective donor should have no pre-existing medical condition, communicable diseases and no major psychiatric illness. The entire process of retrieval of kidneys and subsequent transplantation requires coordinated team effort of one or two different hospitals. Cadaver kidney transplantation can only be performed at an approved transplant centre by NOTTO and hence it is available in hospitals of mostly metropolitan cities.

The selection criteria of both prospective recipient and suitable donor are followed as per NOTTO guidelines, the operative procedure, medication/

immunosuppression etc. are identical to live transplantation and functioning of grafts may not be instant and may take three days to a few weeks to attain optimum functional status. The long-term survival rate in India remains restricted to 1–10 years. Thus, the number of cadaver transplantations remains small. According to estimates of NOTTO, only 840 cadaver transplantations have been undertaken since 1995 in this country of billions.

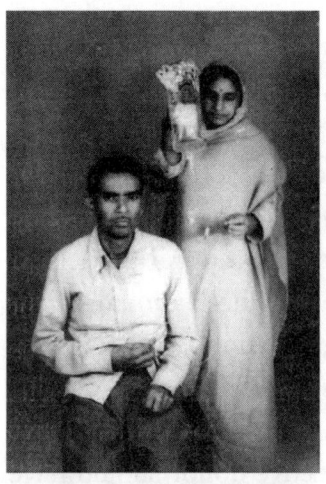

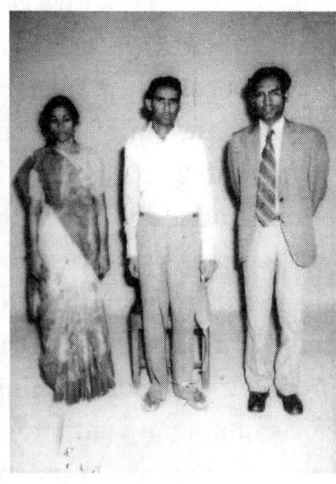

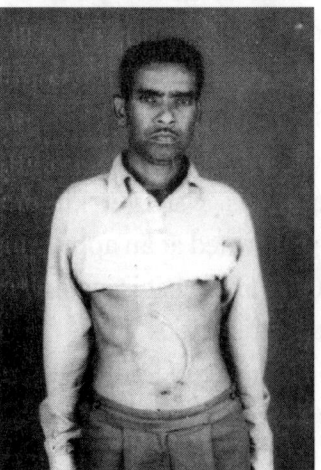

Dr Ramesh Kumar with the first patient who had a CAPD procedure at AIIMS in 1979. This patient was a young man called Devi Das, who did not have a donor and, therefore, became eligible for the CAPD.

PUSHING FOR AN ORGAN TRANSPLANT LAW

I HAD PERSONALLY PROPOSED THE necessity of a Transplantation Act to the Union Health Minister, Dr Karan Singh, at the Annual Convocation at the All India Institute of Medical Sciences, New Delhi in 1974 – some 45 years ago.

For twenty years, no progress took place and the country became an infamous hunting ground for live kidneys for transplantation by the rich across the world in the 1970s and '80s. For nephrologists and surgeons alike, the lawlessness became a shameful scene.

As a senior nephrologist in the country's capital city, I felt the onus was on me to do something about this. Since Members of Parliament were approachable in Delhi, when an opportunity was available or self-created, some of us approached a few Members of the Parliament, Ministers and Union Ministers for approval of a Kidney Transplant Bill in the Lok Sabha, India's lower house of parliament. This was in the early nineties and there was a new government and new health minister in office by then.

My colleague, Dr RVS Yadav, a transplant surgeon, and I were able to see the then Union Health Minister, and he was apprised of the urgent need for the passage of this Bill in the Parliament. *We both were stunned by the most uncaring comment on the proposed legislation, that this practice of 'buying and selling' kidneys was mutually beneficial to both parties.* We felt shocked and thoroughly defeated.

Subsequently, Atal Bihari Vajpayee, the then prominent Member of Parliament was approached, who unhesitatingly accepted our proposition and our argument and pursued the legislation with passion.

Like so many other bills in India's parliament, in the coming years, The Human Organ Transplant Bill was listed in the proceedings of Lok Sabha on a few occasions but could not be discussed.

The Secretary General of Rajya Sabha, the senate, Sudarshan Agarwal, was then approached to see if this legislation could be routed through the Rajya Sabha, the upper house of parliament. He was pleased to assisst us and had this legislation listed for discussion enthusiastically. It was subsequently approved by a majority vote in the Rajya Sabha. The then Vice President, Shankar Dayal Sharma, the Chairman of Rajya Sabha, signed this legislation instantly.

Later, due to the sole efforts of Atal Bihari Vajpayee, the Bill was placed in the Lok Sabha on one late evening and was approved as an Act by a majority vote of available Members of Parliament, that day in July 1994. With assent of the President, THOA came to be passed on the 8th of July 1994. It was added to the statute book as the Transplantation of Human Organs Act, 1994 (the 42nd of 1994). It came into force in the States of Goa, Himachal Pradesh and Maharashtra and all the Union Territories on 4 February 1995.

> **RAJYA SABHA**
>
> **SUPPLEMENT TO THE SYNOPSIS OF DEBATES**
>
> (Proceedings other than Questions & Answers)
>
> Wednesday, May 5, 1993/Vaisakha 15, 1915 (Saka)
>
> **THE TRANSPLANTATION OF HUMAN ORGANS BILL, 1993**
> —Contd.
>
> SHRI JOHN F. PERNANDES: It is mentioned in the Bill that the three States, Goa, Maharashtra and Himachal Pradesh and UTs will implement this Bill. The spirit behind this Bill is very noble. It will protect the nation on human dignity. At the moment, 60 per cent people are living below the poverty line. They are very poor. Just to get their daily meals, they can do anything. They can donate their blood and sell their organs. The anti-social elements take advantage of this situation. Government should request all the States to ensure that this law is implemented. It should be uniformly implemented throughout the country.
>
> The State Governments should be directed to ensure that they should have the Authorisation Committee at the District level. The authorities should be stationed in the State and not in Delhi so that this law may be made more meaningful. The hon. Minister has laid down a penalty for violation of this Act which is 5 years imprisonment or Rs. 10,000. No minimum penalty has been laid down. I feel the law should be made more stringent. There were reports that human beings are exported in the form of adoption. This Bill doesn't cover this aspect. This heinous practice should be stopped by bringing some other legislation. Government should take some precautions to see that there is a ban on the transplantation of the organs which are infected by HIV and AIDS. I support this Bill.
>
> DR. BAPU KALDATE: I feel that there will be a slogan in future—'Transplant your organs. Do not burn or bury them because they are useful.' I am afraid that even after passing this Bill, there may be legal fraud in collecting the human organs. This should be
>
> 104

> 105
>
> seriously considered. Sometime back an article was published in Illustrated Weekly about a village, wherein it was said that the residents of the village were engaged in the trade of human organs.
>
> Goa, Himachal Pradesh, Maharashtra and Union Territory of Delhi have passed this Bill. But this trade will continue in the remaining States. I feel that all the States should pass this Bill so that it may prove effective. Government should refer the Bill to a Select Committee in order to have the opinion of the experts. In principle I welcome the Bill but its shortcomings should be looked into and a comprehensive Bill should be brought.
>
> SHRI SUNIL BASU RAY: This Bill will be applicable to the States and the Union Territories mentioned in it only and for all other places, to make it applicable, a resolution will have to be adopted by the respective State Governments. This aspect should be considered by the Government. To stop private business and profiteering in transplantation of human organs there should be a check by the Government. It should be mentioned as to which hospitals are authorised for the transplantation and storage of human organs. This Bill authorises any medical practitioner for performing such operations. A suitable person must be a surgical man, trained in this particular field. So, the term 'medical practitioner' should also be defined to state clearly as to which medical practitioner, which surigcal person will be authorised to do so. In our country, the storage capacity for such purposes is very less. So, this capacity, should be developed.
>
> The Government should take these points into consideration and bring an amended Bill before us and assure the House that this legislation will be applied throughout India at the same time.
>
> DR. NARREDDY THULASI REDDY: Every year, lakhs of people die because of damage to one or the other organs. So, the transplantation of these organs through the new technology will save the lives of lakhs of people. But unfortunately on the one side, lakhs of people are dying and on the other this illegal trade in transplantation of organs is going on. So, this Bill will serve both the purposes. This Bill curbs the illegal trade as well as it saves the lives of lakhs of people who are dying because of damage to the organs. I support this Bill. The provision of 48 hours is not proper in respect of transplantation of cornea. It should be removed within six hours. There should be a suitable amendment to this provision. So far as accident victims

are concerned, in the person's driving licence itself, there should be a organ donor stamp, along with his blood group. The States will have to ratify this Bill. The mass media should be utilised for creating awareness among the public to donate their organs. There should be some machinery for effective implementation of this law.

SHRI MOOLCHAND MEENA: I support this Bill. The Government should implement this Bill throughout the country at the same time. If it is implemented throughout the country it will have a check on such persons, who are involved in the trade of human organs and who force the poor to sell their organs by alluring them. It should have also been provided that the organs of unclaimed bodies, found at public places, can also be taken out and utilised. The punishment for the misuse of human organs is very less. No one would have dared to misuse it if death penalty would have been prescribed for such an offence.

The sub-clause concerning offences by companies should be removed. This Bill will inspire people to donate their organs. It would provide help to donors to donate their organs at registered centres only. So this Bill should be implemented strictly.

SHRI G. G. SWELL: One of the main objects of the Bill is to prevent commercial deals in human organs. I would like to know whether Government has an idea to have a bank of the human organs in the country because this is a very technical area. India is a poor country in which many people have to sell their organs in order to support themselves and their families. Some day somebody may die. Therefore, we should make some kind of a deal in this regard. A person can donate his eyes when he is strong enough to live for years. In the event of his death his eyes should be removed and preserved for transplantation. Would Government have this kind of a practice in the country when anybody willingly agrees to donate his organs when he is living? Government should create facilities in the country to preserve these organs because there will be hundreds of people who are willing to donate them.

THE MINISTER OF HEALTH AND FAMILY PLANNING (SHRI B. SHANKARANAND), replying to the debate, said: There should not be an indiscriminate transplantation only with monetary interest which leads to undesirable commercial practices. It will be our endeavour to persuade the other States and I am sure they will also fall in line in adopting this Bill. This Bill is brought not only to

| PUSHING FOR AN ORGAN TRANSPLANT LAW |

curb malpractices but also to help the people who want organ transplantation. At the moment, let us not be in naste to introduce stricter penal provisions which may come in the way of the enforcement of the provisions of this Bill. There should be some rule which is uniformaly applicable to all concerned. Only those hospitals, which are registered for this purpose, can undertake surgical intervention in transplantation. Every organ has its own limitation or duration of preservation under scientific or medical conditions. So, efforts are made to see that this period is properly utilised and the organs are preserved. Provision of death sentence for the misuse of this medical intervention facility cannot be allowed. We will have to build up storage facilities also. But we are not going to make any distinction between a Government hospital or a private hospital.

The motion for consideration of the Bill was adopted. Clauses etc., as amended, were adopted. The Bills, as amended, was passed.

THE ACT AND AFTERWARDS

The Bill and subsequent Act was an extremely welcome step in the field of nephrology and transplantation. Since it took time to be adopted in different States, there was a period of uncertainty, confusion and negative press in the country. There were inevitable delays in uniform implementation of the Act in all the States of India and some patients felt frustrated about not being able to get a kidney transplant from an *unrelated donor*.

To a certain extent, the Act curbed the trade of human organs and was a major milestone in medical legislation. The importance of a 'heart-beating cadaver' was realised and debated for a successful cadaver kidney/organ harvesting.

For the first time in India, 'brain death' was recognised and allowed doctors to transplant organs from such patients. In this solemn and stream-lined working protocol, a few medical professionals took advantage of their own opinions and the related publicity. Nevertheless, there were news items like 'kidney patients dread law on transplantation' and 'human organ transplant bill unworkable'.

I would die a peaceful man if in the next two decades, this cadaver donor system (permitted 25 years ago) is adopted nation-wide as a public cause in India. One life saves four lives. I reiterate, one person, upon dying, can donate two kidneys and save two patients. It will enable two patients to come off the dialysis machine and make way for two more patients.[1]

Ever since the Human Organs Transplantation Act was promulgated in India, the transplantation of kidneys, livers, corneas and other human organs is carried out under the guidelines of the Act. Cases of close relation donors are scrutinised and approved

---

[1] India's death rate is about 7 per 1000. Based on this, 8.4 million people die every year in India which comes to 22,500 per day approximately.

by in-house Competent Authority of the approved transplant centres.

The law envisages that all patients needing transplantation other than in cases of genetically-near relatives (including spouses, grandparents, parents, siblings, children and grandchildren, above the age of eighteen years) require a written permission from the State, District-level or Hospital-based Authorisation Committee. The unrelated individuals include even brothers-in-law, sisters-in-law, mother-in-law, father-in-law and immediate cousins.

When the donor is not a near relative and is donating one kidney for reason of affection, attachment and other special reasons, each donor is supposed to be carefully scrutinised and the hospital-based authorisation committee has to approve the donation under strict guidelines prescribed in the Act.

In case the donor is a woman, greater precaution has to be taken and her identity and independent consent has to be confirmed by a person other than the recipient and not under pressure of her husband or other members of family (as many cases of dowry-related and sale of wife's /daughter-in-law's organ has come to light in the past half a century).

SECTION 22 OF THOA

This Section specifically stipulates that the Authorisation Committee shall evaluate and determine that:

(i)   There is no commercial transaction.
(ii) Explanation of the link between them.

(iii) Reasons why the donor wishes to donate.
(iv) Documentary evidence of the link, proof that they have lived together.
(v) Old photographs showing the donor and the recipient together.
(vi) There is no middleman or tout involved.
(vii) Financial status of the donor and the recipient, evidence of their vocation and income for the previous three financial years and that there is no gross disparity between the status of the two.
(viii) The donor is not a drug addict.
(ix) Ensure awareness and verify intention to donate kidney, details of surgery involved, authenticity of link between donor and recipient and the reasons for donation or any other views expressed which have to be recorded and taken note of.
(x) Verification of Aadhaar card online and screen shot maintained.
(xi) Verification of issued certificate in respect of domicile status of recipient or donor by speed post.
(xii) Photo ID proof of the person (next of kin) giving consent to the donor.
(xiii) Documents of each transplant be thoroughly scrutinised and signed by the legal cell and the transplant cell of the hospital.
(xiv) ID proof of interpreter/translator shall be verified in each case if required.
(xv) The evaluation of psychological and mental health of a donor is mandatory.

A kidney transplant from an 'unrelated donor' is extremely difficult to organise and is a time-consuming exercise both for donor and recipient. It takes about 2–3 weeks for completion of all documents and formalities in the strictest manner with the help of the transplant coordinator of the hospital. Invariably, the waiting time is rather long, and all unrelated donors and recipients are required to go through a stringent process to establish the genuineness of their relationships and intention to donate a kidney and undergo transplantation.

In spite of all steps fulfilled and approval of the Authorisation Committee sought, a very large grey area of fictitious documentation and impersonation is a common occurrence in most kidney transplant centres in the country. Media does not help.

PUSHING FOR AN ORGAN TRANSPLANT LAW

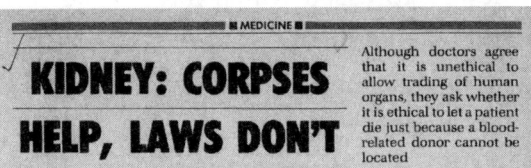

THE YEARS BETWEEN 1994 AND 2004

The next ten years following the passing of the THOA, however, saw places like Gurugram, Noida, Ghaziabad in the National Capital Region as hubs of the kidney trade, and a large number of patients made a queue for newly-sprouting ill-equipped hospitals for transplantation in these areas. Cities like Chennai and Kolkata too emerged as places where anyone could just 'buy' a kidney and get a transplant.

During this interim teething period, the media too was against the Act and published stories of difficulties faced by patients while medical personnel complained about the lack of implementation of the Act. Certain medical professionals took advantage of the mood in the media to get their own opinions published in print and visual media. Despite this, their opinions did not have an expeditious impact on the speedy implication of the Act uniformly across the country.

LEGAL ORGAN DONATION RARE

Even though the THOA came into force in 1995, legal organ donations continue to remain rare in India.

The Multi Organ Harvesting Aid Network (MOHAN) began to spearhead legal organ donation in Chennai in 1997.[2]

---

[2] MOHAN Foundation is a not-for-profit, nongovernmental organisation started to promote organ donation in 1997 in Chennai by philanthropists and medical professionals led by Dr Sunil Shroff. It is a registered NGO with Income Tax exemption under Section 80G and 35AC and has offices in Chennai, Hyderabad, Delhi-NCR, Chandigarh, Nagpur, Jaipur, Mumbai and USA. MOHAN Foundation was started by a group

In India, there are just 1 per million legal cadaver donations. 'On an average, half a million people are dying for the want of organs every year as there is an extreme shortage of organ donation to the patients when they are declared end-stage organ failure', Dr H Jauhari, Chairman Renal Transplant Division, Sir Ganga Ram Hospital and member of National Organ Tissue Transplant Organisation (NOTTO) told ANI on the World Organ Donation Day in August 2019.

As many as 20 per million cadaver organ donation takes place in Spain, US, France and other countries. Not in India, however. This is due to illiteracy, poverty and the presence of money-making touts who take advantage of Indians who don't know better.

PUSHING FOR AN ORGAN TRANSPLANT LAW

---

of like-minded and concerned medical and non-medical professionals committed to increasing the reach of the Transplantation of Human Organs Act. The Government of India passed this act in 1994 to broaden the concept of organ donation and stop commercial dealings in organs, especially kidneys. It is now possible to not only donate one's eyes, but also other vital organs like the heart, lungs, liver, pancreas and kidneys.

https://www.mohanfoundation.org/who.asp

KIDNEY TRANSPLANT IN INDIA

THE FIRST RECORDED HUMAN KIDNEY transplant was performed by Dr Mathieu Jaboulay in Lyon, France.[1] He made the first attempts to transplant kidneys into humans in 1906. He was using goat and pig kidneys, and naturally, the transplants did not work. Transplant science has evolved much since then.

Jaboulay's associate, Alexis Carrel, did pioneering work on the surgical technique of vascular suturing (stitching up the veins) and was awarded the Nobel Prize for his work in 1912.

In the early 1950s, human kidney transplantation was undertaken in Paris, and in December 1954, Dr Joseph E Murray performed the world's first successful human kidney transplant at the Peter Bent Brigham Hospital in Boston, Massachusetts in the United States.

---

[1] https://en.wikipedia.org/wiki/Mathieu_Jaboulay

YEARS OF EFFORT IN INDIA

In India, the first two human kidney transplants were performed at KEM Hospital in Mumbai in May 1965, from cadaver donors. Both patients died, one on the 11th post-operative day with a functional graft, and the second patient died on the 3rd post-operative day due to a chest infection.

The first successful 'live donor' kidney transplant in India was performed at the CMC Vellore by Dr Mohan Rao and Dr KV Johny on 2nd February 1971.

Though this was almost 17 years after the first transplant by Murray in 1954, a successful start had been made in the field of human renal transplantation in India by the Vellore team. They concluded that renal transplantation was *feasible* in India and has a definite future. The Vellor team had, however, warned that inadequately and improperly planned attempts at transplantation might lower the morale of the patients, as well as the public. Since then many thousand transplants have been done in this country, but in the absence of a proper system of registry, it is impossible to ascertain the exact number of transplants done so far in India.

Dr RVS Yadav performed the second successful transplant at the Post Graduate Institute of Medical Sciences and Research (PGI), Chandigarh in June 1973.

The first 'living related' kidney transplant was done at the All India Institute of Medical Sciences (AIIMS, Delhi) in July–August 1973. It fell upon me, as the senior nephrologist at AIIMS, and as one who championed organ transplant, to ensure the most untiring efforts to make this procedure a success.

Incidentally, the second kidney transplant at AIIMS was from an 'unrelated' donor, which was not considered illegal at that point in time in India. When the donor did not return for a follow-up, the family of the recipient disclosed that *a payment was made to the donor* and that he was doing well and did not consider a follow-up to be of any importance.

This transplant, however, was the moment of great exhilaration for my entire team and I, and the institution and it was widely acclaimed in the print media. We were technology pioneers. For us, it was a validation that lives could be saved with donated organs.

The early years of kidney transplantation in India were extremely effort-oriented for nephrology and surgical teams.

The resources were meager, but commitment and enthusiasm were abundant. There were, of course, trying periods of great anxiety and uncertainty of patient recovery and acceptance of the transplanted kidney by the system of the recipient. Supply of immunosuppression agents from pharmaceutcal outlets were limited. For medical personnel, there was immense satisfaction when a patient got better and left the hospital. With limited resources available, maximum efforts were invested concerning the wellbeing of the patient and the kidney donor. The gratitude expressed by the families was rewarding for the nephrologist and surgeon. The whole process did not include greed, and for a successful outcome, motivation was the best ingredient for the transplantation.

PEOPLE'S LEADER JAYAPRAKASH NARAYAN

In the early seventies, the medical fraternity and young pioneers like me in the field of nephrology were striving hard to surmount teething problems of the transplantation process.

In June of 1975, Independence activist and popular political leader Jayaprakash Narayan was detained by the authorities during the infamous 'Emergency' period. After his initial medical checkup in AIIMS, Delhi, JP (as he was popularly known) was moved to the PGI, Chandigarh. Reports say, he was kept for 130 days at the PGI and was released on 12 November 1975.

PGI was in the news in those days for kidney-related treatments.[2]

---

[2] 1. A book by Gyan Prakash describes how JP was brought to Chandigarh on 1 July 1975. He was 73 then. The District Magistrate of Chandigarh, MG Devasahayam, was under instructions from Haryana Chief Minister Bansi Lal, 'Usko wahin pade rehne do. Kisi se milne ya telephone mat karne dena. Apne aap ko hero samajhta hai'.

Devasahayam's narrative offers an account of JP's despondency: 'I wonder what use my life is going to be in captivity. Everything seems to be finished.' The fiery revolutionary was going through a low, having lost his wife Prabhawati some time before.

JP's health deteriorated during his four months of captivity in Chandigarh.

Later, at Jaslok Hospital in Bombay, he was found to be suffering from kidney ailments.

The book says that 'the conduct of the doctors at PGI, led by the redoubtable Dr PN Chuttani, did not breed confidence, in view of Bansi Lal's attitude'. MG Devasahayam, now living in Nagercoil, near Kanyakumari down South, says, he found the doctors' attitude 'grey'.

When Jayaprakash Narayan arrived at AIIMS, Delhi from Chandigarh late one evening of November 1975, I examined him and found that he was grossly fluid-overloaded, with swelling in his legs, face and congestion in his chest. He was suffering from long-standing diabetes mellitus and was treated with conservative treatment, fluid restriction and diuretics (to increase urine output). His kidney function tests showed that they were not functioning properly. I, therefore, concluded that Jayaprakashji was in need of urgent hemodialysis.

His complete medical investigations were done without publicity, as I was instructed to work in complete privacy by the administration and an emissary of the then Prime Minister, Indira Gandhi.

I was asked to wait before communicating even with JP's brother Rajeshwar Prasad and was told to remain at home and to expect a call from the office of the Prime Minister, regarding JP. To my great surprise, Prime Minister Indira Gandhi herself spoke to me and was apprised of the urgent need of

---

2. Devasahayam says: Mysteriously in early November 1975, JP's health started deteriorating fast and from doctor's hedgy replies about his health, 'I suspected that something was amiss. As later events proved, JP's kidney was getting irrevocably damaged! Under the circumstances, I was convinced that it would be unsafe to keep JP in Chandigarh any longer and he should get to a place where his ailment could be diagnosed correctly and treated properly.'
https://www.tribuneindia.com/news/chandigarh/jp-atpgi-history-in-your-backyard/697656.html
https://www.thehinducentre.com/the-arena/currentissues/article25188707.ece

3. Devasahayam has extensively discussed JP's detention and health in his two books with Vitasta: *Jaiprakash ki Aakhri Jail* (Hindi) and *JP Movement: Emergency and India's Second Freedom.*

hemodialysis. I had, naturally, also kept Rajeshwar Prasadji informed of JP's condition.

I was then asked to talk to Jayaprakash Narayan's brother and inform him that JP needed further treatment and hemodialysis. I was told to suggest that this was preferably to be carried out in Mumbai. It was a very sensitive situation in a charged environment, and the family moved him to Jaslok Hospital in Mumbai. Thus, JP was kept away from Delhi, the national capital and the heart of India's political activity at that time.

On 25 February 1977, I read a long narration in the *Times of India* newspaper in which it was alleged that JP's kidneys were damaged deliberately in the course of treatment during detention in Chandigarh. This was very disheartening to read. To even imagine that a prestigious national medical institution can be pressurised and politically coerced to 'deliberately' damage a famous detainee's kidneys and that well-known nephrologists providing care would become those who actually inflict damage on a old man in their care is completely demoralising for the entire profession.[3]

---

[3] http://pgimer.edu.in/PGIMER_PORTAL/PGIMERPORTAL/home.jsp

KIDNEY SCAMS IN INDIA

MY REMINISCENCE TAKES ME BACK to 1963 when, as a young medical student, I was unable to recognise a pathology specimen of kidney instantly.

With a pause I was able to recite the entire description and causes of 'a large white kidney in a large white man'. It rekindled a fire in me, fueling me to obtain all the laurels of the undergraduate period in the university.

Later, as the junior-most resident doctor in the medicine department, it was painful each time when my professor would just pass by a case of uremia (chronic renal disease) – such were the distressful feelings in me in the mid-sixties. With singular effort, I was able to reach a unit in the UK, where procedure of dialysis used to take 14 hours each time on a patient on maintenance hemodialysis.

In this world of multiplying wonders, the creation of artificial organs and transplantation of organs, capable of prolonging and sustaining optimum health is one of the most spectacular feats.

Kidney transplantation was also beginning across hospitals in the United Kingdom and it was the greatest opportunity for me to explore in the field of nephrology and organ transplantation. It was an atmosphere all-around of great satisfaction for those involved in this field and there were no stresses in the social milieu.

After my graduation (MBBS) in 1964 and MD (Medicine) in 1967, I did an MRCP (Renal) in 1971. I was appointed as Assistant Professor (Renal and Electrolyte) to develop the specialty of Nephrology and Transplantation at AIIMS, Delhi. Dr KK Malhotra was appointed Associate Professor of Medicine with an interest in the department of Renal and Electrolyte. After a few months of my joining AIIMS, at this crucial time, when the nephrology department was just beginning to take shape, Dr Malhotra decided to move to Ahvaz, Iran for two years. The entire responsibility of developing 'specialty and service of nephrology' and transplantation then rested on me. Thus, for fourteen years, I became the face of the AIIMS nephrology department, and this continued until I chose to move out of AIIMS in 1984.

In India, the scene was similar to the UK in the early seventies. A platform existed for experimentation and innovation in an academic hospital setting. Soon, however, the number of patients seeking dialysis and kidney transplantation became extremely high in all centres where such facilities were available.

The unending queues of patients with kidney failure and very large number of patients coming from different parts of Northern India seeking treatment was a tremendous load on my working schedule in AIIMS as a specialist each day. This had put an extremely heavy pressure on me, and I started feeling that my commitment to renal medicine was becoming less as the years were passing.

This feeling engulfed me and I had started to become restless. I was not contributing anything to medicine and study, to research and innovation, I felt. A time soon came when I was clear that the only way out was to leave the prestigious mecca of medical education, training of medical man-power and patient care. I had no doubt that I had to continue to practice for what I was determined and committed to in my entire life – developments and progress in the field of nephrology.

The plight of poor patients and the helplessness of their families and most, of their spouses, is still vivid in front of my eyes and unfortunately the entire scene in the vast country has not changed, and it still haunts me.

EXPANDING SERVICES

My mission in the 14 years at AIIMS had included creating identical departments at Sir Ganga Ram Hospital, New Delhi and kidney centres at Jaipur, Agra, Lucknow and Kanpur. Similar centres and facilities were also developing in other places across the country. By the 1980s, transplantation facilities were available in major cities such as Bombay, Madras, Hyderabad, Calcutta, Chandigarh and Ahmedabad.

The fraternity of nephrologists in the country were busy defining the patterns of kidney diseases and kidney failures of acute and chronic types and practices of dialysis and transplantation. A large number of patients seeking dialysis were refused at most centres for the lack of available treatment space. There were few centres and facilities for transplantation, and the awareness to seek dialysis and transplantation was minimal.

There were only two immunosuppressive drugs – Prednisolone and Azathioprine. Later, in the eighties, the availability of Cyclosporine enhanced the success and longevity of kidney transplants.

In the absence of any legislation, the practice of kidney transplantation was without any hurdles. The so called 'cousins' as donors were readily accepted all over the country and, there were no scandals and scams in kidney transplantation.

The majority of kidney donors were from families, but the wealthy patients and patients with no similar donor blood group in their families looked for donors from unrelated sources.

During this period, such kidney transplantations were not considered to be an unholy practice. Word of mouth and success stories in the media contributed for preferential availability of unrelated kidney donors. The close-knit family structure with high emotional bondage had contributed to seeking donors from outside sources. The medical fraternity had also contributed with their advice to seek donors from outside in selected cases of those with strong family history of diabetes etc. The care and follow-up of successful kidney transplant patient was satisfactory in those days, and the majority were from within the cities or nearby towns, resulting in a small number of total cases in the country. A few patients from neighbouring countries like Nepal and Afghanistan came to AIIMS, Chandigarh and CMC Vellore, the two centres that were at that time internationally known.

In the seventies, there was no cadaveric transplantation facility available in the country, and this alternative was never considered by kidney physicians or transplant surgeons. Nephrologists were at the forefront of advice and treatment modalities and were responsible for taking decisions in transplantation activities. Till that time, the transplant surgeons remained confined just to the surgical practice and care of patients.

The financial assistance from government sources was always insufficient to support the treatment of a patient and, therefore, the entire burden of kidney-related expenses was on the patients themselves.

Sociologically speaking, by the 1980s, the kidney cure scene deteriorated rapidly and soon became painful. Young married women were the worst victims and the future of children got compromised. The medical personnel had no time to perceive or interact with this aspect of cure management.

Long-term hemodialysis was not within financial reach of most patients, and only a few were able to opt for kidney transplantation with large expenditure at one time. The expense was often met by taking loans or disposing of fixed assets. Sustaining a newly-acquired life at any cost overrode the hurdles of financial burdens, the poor became poorer and people just above the poverty-line slumped below it.

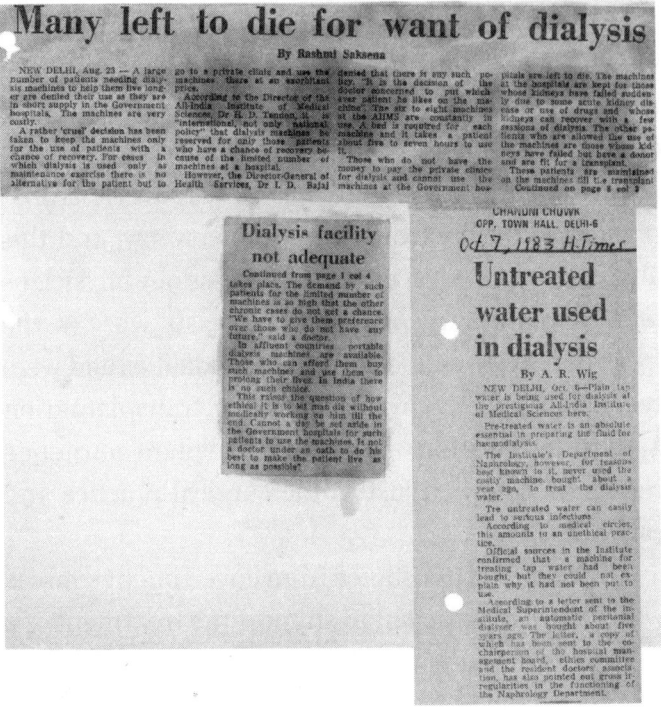

KIDNEY SCAMS IN INDIA

PURCHASED AND UNRELATED

The second transplant at AIIMS, New Delhi and an early case at CMC, Vellore were from unrelated sources – the donors were paid undisclosed amounts of money by the families of the recipients.

With the practice of kidney transplantation, having once started and accepted, in the '80s, India became a kidney bazaar. In the absence of prescribed guidelines and legislation at the time, the practice of kidney transplantation was not uniform across the country. Most transplant centres followed their own protocol and treatment plans including different immunosuppression regimens. The formations of the Indian Society of Nephrology (ISN) and the Indian Society of Organ Transplantation (ISOT) were in early stages and until the late nineties, practical guidelines for kidney transplantation were different at each transplant centre.

TYPES OF DONORS

Cousin Donors: In the early stages of transplantation, any suitable family members including first- and second-degree relatives were accepted as kidney donors.

There was open solicitation of donors in the media, along with advertisements in public places like railway stations, bazaars, cinema halls.

A perceptible change in the scene of kidney transplantation happened when 'unrelated paid donors' appeared in the garb of being 'cousins' of the prospective recipient and the practice gradually spread throughout the country. As the availability of such kidney donor became possible, families of the recipients began to prefer obtaining a kidney from outside sources.

Professional Blood Donors: It had been a common practice to tap professional blood donors for compatible blood requirement on payment. In the past, these victims were lured into kidney donation on the promise of lucrative payments. Unfortunately, most of these donors were malnourished, anemic and carriers of diseases. In this trade, kidney brokers, doctors, laboratories and hospitals had actively participated as there was no check on these 'kidney merchants'. The professional blood donors were mostly drug addicts as well those who were in dire need of money. While frequent blood donation once or twice in a week would fetch only a few hundred rupees which would end up in country liquor dens, earning a large amount of many thousands to lakhs of rupees appeared a much more lucrative proposition to these people.

There was an unprecedented uproar by the media, the courts, prominent individuals of society, NGOs, the administration, the police, the ministries of Home Affairs, Health and Family Welfare in May 1992 following the exposure of a kidney removal for transplantation in a private hospital in the capital city of India, where the donor was a drug addict.

Self-soliciting Donors: The practice of self-solicitation to sell or buy a kidney had no hurdles or checks in open trade of human organs during the eighties and nineties. There were advertisements in the media by donors and recipients with explicit details of blood group, address, age with offers of suitable rewards. There was direct communication by willing donors to sell their kidney to doctors and I myself have received many such letters in the eighties and early nineties. There was a complete lull in this practice soon after THOA was made a law in May 1994. Today one hears of such sporadic news items and as usual, no real action is taken.

Altruistic Donors: This category, permitted in the THOA 1994, was used as a loophole by middlemen exploiting impoverished individuals. Touts would bribe administrative authorisation committees or coach unrelated donors and manipulate images to make it seem like the recipient and donor were connected.

Unrelated Donors, through Financial Incentives: The experiment of 'gift rewarding' through hospital at Guest Hospital, Chennai in the nineties had failed and had not received acceptance in the country and worldwide. It was full of lacunae and considered devoid of ethics. Dr KC Reddy has quoted in one of his articles that those against paid organ transplantation condemn this practice as 'victimisation of the poor, a form of corporeal prostitution, resonant with the undertones of slavery'.

Unrelated Donors, by Coercion or Deceit: As family structures are shifting to nuclear, in a male-dominated family system, the brunt of any illness is borne by the female members of a family.

There are frequent reports even today of marriages arranged to poor women to acquire a kidney for an already ailing husband whose illness is willingly concealed. There are instances where a young female is misdiagnosed for an abdominal illness and in a surgical procedure of laparotomy a kidney is removed for transplantation. In a gruesome scene newly-married young wife and widowed women are emotionally pressured to donate a kidney without much information and the consent is obtained by fraudulent means.

In the early days of transplants in India, the practice of hemodialysis and kidney transplantation were considered highly skilled jobs and the concerned doctors greatly esteemed by all. The transplant surgeons and nephrologists were recipients of social accolades and academic recognitions of high standard. At that time, participation of private institutions was negligible, and, in the seventies, centres were confined to government hospitals only. Such was the scene of transplantation in the seventies, in which medical personnel were busy doing their best for the patients and striving all the time to publish their work and the result of their efforts.

KIDNEY SCAMS IN INDIA

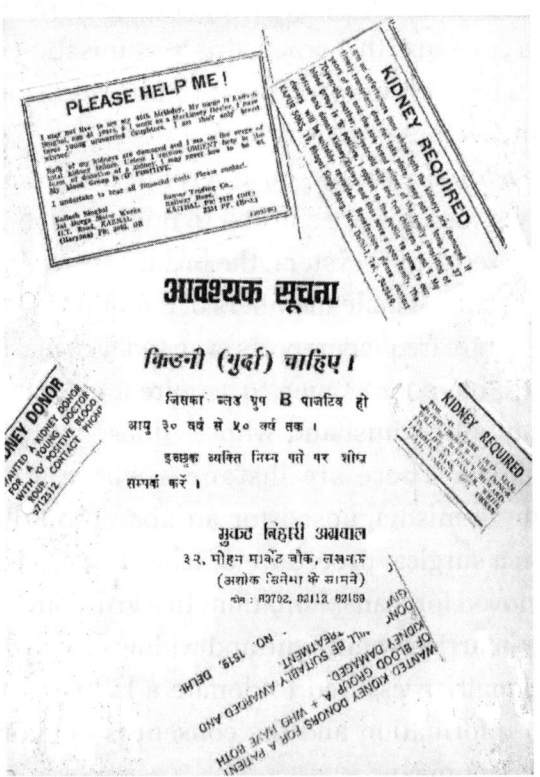

This is the way newspapers carried offers from volunteers trying to sell their kidneys.

INDIA BECOMES THE WORLD'S KIDNEY BAZAAR

THE COMMERCE OF ORGAN HARVESTING became well established across the nation in the 1980s.

The legislative and executive officers of the country had no inkling of the gravity of this illegal trade, and all efforts made by people such as myself remained futile.

During the eighties and nineties, the practice of kidney transplantation grew in all metropolitan cities like Mumbai (hospitals including Jaslok Hospital, Breach Candy Hospital, Cumballa Hill and Bhatia Hospital), Pune, Chennai, Kolkata, Bengaluru, Ahmadabad, Hyderabad, Chandigarh and Delhi (hospitals including AIIMS, Batra Hospital, Sir Ganga Ram Hospital, and the Army Hospital).

CHANGING SCENE OF KIDNEY TRANSPLANTATION

There was open soliciting of kidney donors in print media across the country, and unscrupulous individuals soon began to mediate on behalf of the recipient with cash offers to prospective kidney donors.

There were advertisements in newspapers with exhaustive details of the desired blood group, address, desirable age and details of their young families, including suitable rewards to make it a complete racket.

There were, often, even postings made by prospective kidney donors offering to sell their own organs. At the time, there were no hurdles or checks on this open trade of human organs across the country. Posters of 'kidney donor' and 'kidney required' were pasted in public places like cinema halls, railway stations, and even on lamp posts.

As the number of transplant centres gradually increased, the availability of kidney donors increased – donors shifted from being relatives of the recipient to solicited groups.

However, as the trend of purchased kidneys grew, the medical fraternity began to suspect these so-called 'cousins', even though they were presented by the recipient family themselves. There were just a few middlemen involved in the early stages, and this was the beginning of a different scene in medicine where payments and donations to such unrelated donors became a norm. This soon led to increasing exploitation of the poor. Their kidneys could be purchased.

At the same time, with the availability of better immunosuppressive agents that contained rejection by the recipient body, the spouses of recipients with similar blood groups became increasingly acceptable as suitable donors. This again resulted in several tragedies. One incident I was witness to unravelled like this:

> In this tragic episode, a man of thirty-six years had been on biweekly hemodialysis for nearly one year and had no suitable kidney donor as both, his mother and father, had diabetes. His younger brother was not prepared to donate a kidney.
>
> His wife was of similar blood group but she too was reluctant to donate her kidney as she had two children to care for. Ultimately, the wife was persuaded by the family to donate a kidney to the husband.
>
> The woman underwent a complete nephrological investigation. For some reason, the woman's parents were not available throughout the preparation phase and it was a situation of non-availability of next of kin for the woman.
>
> Both husband and wife, under oath, had produced an affidavit under the signature of the city magistrate and the transplant operation was scheduled for a particular date.
>
> The woman's recipient husband was admitted two days before the transplant operation and the following day, his donor wife was supposed to check in to the transplant centre.
>
> However, she did not appear in the hospital and went on telling her husband on the phone that she was making arrangements to leave their children with her parents.
>
> The whole day passed by waiting, and ultimately, she did not appear for hospital admission and the transplant operation was indefinitely postponed.
>
> We doctors at the hospital later learned that she had moved out to her parents' house with her children.

For the young man, the tragic end came six months later when he was admitted at a very critical stage with high fever and systemic infection and ultimately died in spite of all treatment. Painfully, the wife had not even made an appearance in the last four-five days of her husband's illness, did not come to see the dying husband.

INDIA BECOMES THE WORLD'S KIDNEY BAZAAR

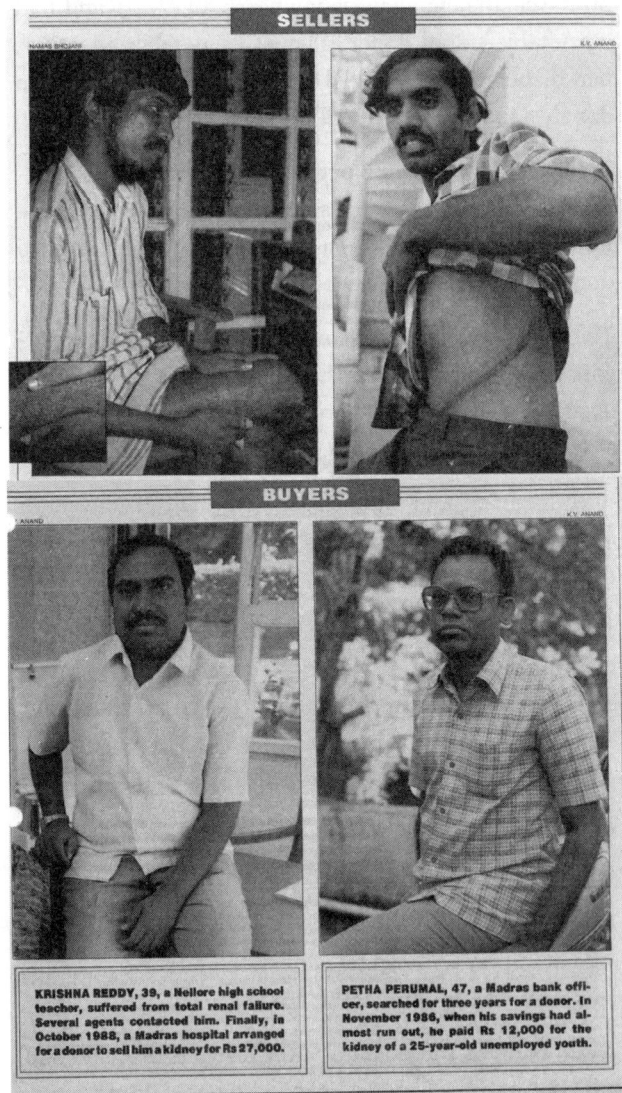

SELLERS

BUYERS

KRISHNA REDDY, 39, a Nellore high school teacher, suffered from total renal failure. Several agents contacted him. Finally, in October 1988, a Madras hospital arranged for a donor to sell him a kidney for Rs 27,000.

PETHA PERUMAL, 47, a Madras bank officer, searched for three years for a donor. In November 1986, when his savings had almost run out, he paid Rs 12,000 for the kidney of a 25-year-old unemployed youth.

Two decades after the first transplant in India, the practice of kidney transplantation was widespread across the country. But there is no dearth of depressing stories either. It is not only wives who chicken out of organ donation, I have even witnessed a mother refusing to save her son.

> A young man in late 20s, whose life was sustained on biweekly hemodialysis in Jaipur, Rajasthan had come to AIIMS in Delhi for kidney transplantation. His mother was his kidney donor.
>
> All investigations and treatment were undertaken as outpatients for the son and mother as they had limited finances and told us they had collected money for the operation by selling their house and land in the native village. We, therefore, did not admit them in the hospital and provided them with all the support services as outpatients.
>
> Just two days before the date of the kidney transplantation, we were told that part of the money against the sale of their property had not been paid by the purchaser and whatever small quantity of jewellery they had in the family was sold in the gold shop outside the All India Institute of Medical Sciences (AIIMS). Their funds, were, thus limited. We still hoped to do the transplant on the young patient as planned.
>
> This family, thus, lost their home and small holding of land. After this, the fate of this young patient became more cruel when his mother became hostile and refused to give her kidney to save his life.
>
> In spite of all medical reasoning by our team and persuasion by her husband (the young man's father) the mother ran away from the hospital. Her argument was – that she had three more children to look after in her life.

I have no follow up except painful remembrance of this episode in my professional life.

Ironically, this gold shop and few other such gold shops continue to function even today and do roaring business on the plight of poor patients coming for treatment in big hospitals, including just outside premier national institutions like the AIIMS.

We at the nephrology department were witness to yet another strange case, I recall. This was after the Transplant Act came into force.

> A brother and sister were the donor and recipient in this case and we at the hospital were relieved at the chance of performing a successful transplant, without having to worry about matching an unrelated donor.
>
> In this well-matched kidney transplant operation, the kidney donor was an older brother to a young lady who was going to be the recipient. All hospital protocol and all provisions of the Transplantation Act were complied with. Suddenly, a team of two policemen had appeared in the hospital a day before the scheduled transplant date with an arrest warrant for the prospective donor brother.
>
> We found out that the police had come to arrest the brother on a complaint of bigamy by his wife. She had alleged that a court had not granted the couple the divorce the man had sought. Nevertheless, while he was married to her still, he had married another woman and had concealed this fact from his family.
>
> So, the hospital foyer turned into a venue of high commotion of shouting and denials. The participants to this emotional outburst were the two families – of the recipient sister and of the proposed kidney donor brother. Amidst this ruckus waited the police, handcuffs ready. The

operation was eventually indefinitely postponed, and the fate of future events remain unknown to the medical team.

Meanwhile, organ commerce kept stride with the advance in medicine.

The commercial trade and exploitation of the poor was rampant, and the Organ Transplant Act had not yet been promulgated by the Government of India. There was an aggressive debate among the medical fraternity for and against buying kidneys – hospitals began to think in terms of rewarding and gifting donors, transparent screenings and stopping unrelated kidney transplantation completely.

Why?...Why not?

WHEN kidney transplants started in the early 1970s, only related (from blood relatives) donor transplants were possible. With the introduction of immuno-suppressive drugs (which suppress the body's mechanism to reject foreign material) like Cyclosporine, both cadaver and unrelated donor transplants became possible.

Cadaver transplants (the donated organ is taken from the body of a clinically dead person) are not yet legally sanctioned in India. Doctors are divided on the question of allowing cadaver transplants, both on ethical and technical grounds. However, the section insisting that brain death (that terminal stage when recovery is medically impossible) be made the criterion for cadaver transplants seems to be gaining in support, both from patients and scientists.

Even if a law allowing cadaver transplants is passed, problems may arise if relatives of a dead person who had donated his organs object to their being removed on religious or other grounds. Besides, the law may even encourage unscrupulous doctors to certify clinically alive patients as dead. There is, after all, a lot of money waiting to be made.

MAXIMUM CITY MUMBAI KIDNEY TRADE EPICENTRE

IT DID NOT TAKE LONG for the city of Mumbai to turn into the biggest centre of organ trade in the country as the city had several competent hospitals offering transplant services.

One senior nephrologist at Bombay Hospital, in an article for *India Today*, wrote in 1990, 'we are burying our heads in the sand'.

'What does one do when there are no organs forthcoming from cadavers? Do I turn my patient away and say prepare for your death? As long as it is properly regulated there is nothing wrong with organ transplants.'

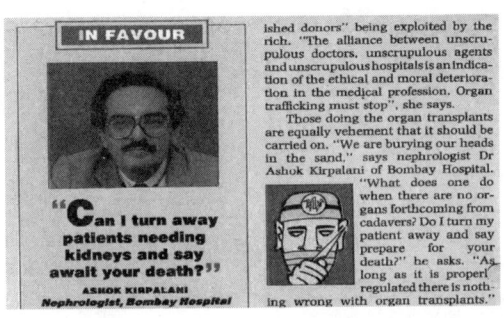

India Today, 31 July 1990.

At the same time, some hospitals employed an illconceived approach to try to break the grip of middlemen by starting to advertise for kidneys themselves.

A new term was coined – reward gifting.[1] Here, unrelated donors completed paperwork including affidavits attesting 'deep love and affection' for the patient.

This led to a storm of counter-arguments from much of the medical fraternity and hospitals that had already stopped transplantation from unrelated kidney donors. This resulted in an 'illegal' trade that quickly spread to private nursing homes in the suburbs of Mumbai and neighbouring cities like Pune.

Surgeries were often performed in temporary clinics without licenses and there were many reports of serious post-operative complications in ill-equipped nursing homes, *where at least a few donors lost their lives*. There was no check on pre-operative screening of hepatitis-B or HIV among donors, and subsequent complications were largely ignored and forgotten. The police and Maharashtra State Medical Council struggled to put an end to the problem.

Mumbai became a preferred destination for patients seeking paid kidney donors, particularly among Arab countries. Proximity to India's west coast was not the only reason. At that time, Mumbai was India's richest city, its commercial hub.

---

[1] Two doctors, Thiagarajan and Reddy from Guest Hospital in Madras, in August 1989 presented their preliminary observations on results of their first 350 unrelated live donor transplants at a Congress on 'Ethics, Justice and Commerce in Transplantation – A Global Issue' held at Ottawa in Canada and advocated the concept of 'Rewarded Gifting'.

These wealthy Arab patients would get admitted in well-known hospitals such as Breach Candy Hospital and Jaslok Hospital, get dialysis done there. They then received transplantation in private nursing homes. After the transplant, the recipient returned to these hospitals for the post-operative care and treatment. Such patients would stay in hospitals for months, get well, and entire families would come for medical checkups and shopping.

Hospitals provided up-to-date medical care and earned large amounts of money through this trade of transplantation. The doctors and nursing homes made their money without any responsibility of aftercare. In this game of misuse and exploitation, the donor was paid a pittance and shunted out with no mercy from anybody.

This practice quickly moved to cities like Pune and Jaipur. It was estimated that in the early '90s, kidney trade had a turnover of ₹40 crore in Mumbai alone. Soon Bombay had worldwide attention and became a dubious city where kidneys were treated as a marketable commodity.

The role of city laboratories was thoroughly intermixed, and there were several instances of tampering of reports by middlemen.

The concerned doctors too were to be blamed. They were not concerned with rechecking vital reports of the donors before accepting them as a 'related' or 'an altruistic unrelated' donor. Of course, soon the relationship between donor and doctor became totally commercial.

FIRST WORDS OF WARNING

At this juncture came a warning from the International Transplantation Society. It said, 'no doctor shall be involved directly or indirectly in buying or selling of organs for any transplantation activity aimed at commercial gain'. The society warned that any doctor found engaged in commercial organ trade 'will stand expulsion'.

It was an India that had given up all ethics and scientific norms by that time and only money mattered. The country was going through a political crisis, and unstable governments by purchasable legislators were in and out of power. There was acute financial crisis too for the Indian economy and the much-touted Narasimha Rao government's reforms were still to show some effect. The International Transplantation Society's warning had no impact on the kidney trade whatsoever. Despite this warning, the roaring business of brokers, doctors and hospitals continued in Mumbai, and the kidney was the hottest marketable commodity sold anywhere between ₹30,000 to ₹50,000 apiece.

The indigent donor was in desperate need of hard cash, and there was always a rich buyer available with the help of a broker, sub-broker, doctors and hospitals. Even senior doctors needing such transplants had no qualms about 'purchasing' kidneys for themselves.

It also became a prevalent practice of random donors writing letters to practicing nephrologists, transplant surgeons and even hospitals directly to sell their kidney and bypass the brokerage and harassment by brokers.

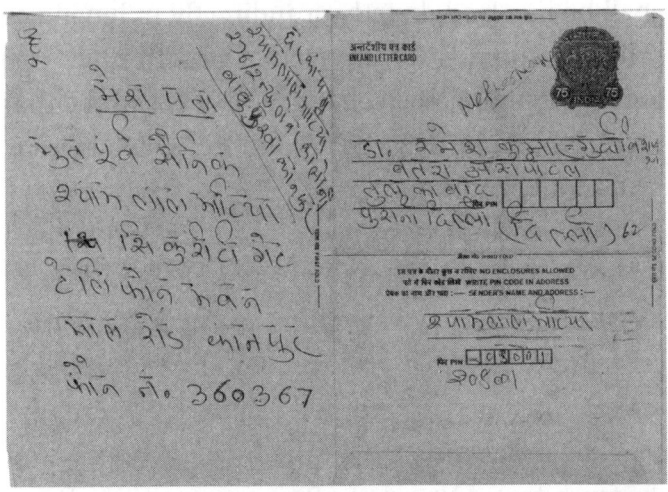

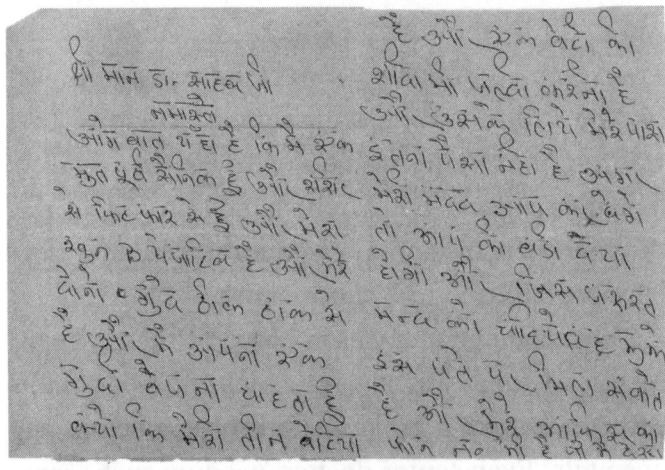

MAXIMUM CITY MUMBAI KIDNEY TRADE EPICENTRE

This letter came from a retired soldier, who was so poor that he wanted to sell his kidney.

डॉ. साहब मेरे Kidney donate करने से एक पंथ से काज की स्थिति यदि तो चरितार्थ हो ही है। एक, तो मेरे परिवार को पुनः नया जीवन मिल जायेगा और दूसरी जिस व्यक्ति को Kidney की आवश्यकता होगी उसकी जिंदगी भी तो बच जायेगी।

जहाँ तक मेरी जानकारी के अनुसार जीवित अंगों के लेन-देन के धंधे में लगे agents के घोखा-धड़ी के भी कई मामले आपको भी ज्ञात होंगे ही।

अतः इस पत्र में लिखी बातें आप उन agents तक नहीं जाने दिजियेगा, अन्यथा हो सकता है कि "मैं अपना जीवन भी व्यर्थ गंवाऊं और मुझे पैसे भी न मिले और मेरा परिवार भी तबाह हो जाये।" कृपया आप इस बात का ध्यान रखियेगा।

कृपया आप अति शीघ्र पत्र लिखकर मेरी समस्या का समाधान कीजिए। Check up की जब भी आवश्यकता होगी मैं आने को तैयार हूँ। यह भी हो सकता है कि मेरे Kidney donate करने के बाद भी मैं जीवित रहूं, तो फिर इसमें परेशानी ही क्या है। डॉ. साहब जरा सोचिये कि तो मरीज मेरी जगह आप होते तो शायद आपको भी ऐसी ही कुर्बानी देनी पड़ती, इसलिए आप मेरे मन की व्यथा को समझने की कोशिश कीजिए और यह कार्य होना ही चाहिए।

धन्यवाद।

My Address
S.K. Vidyarthi C/o
G.C. Ram, R.T.S.
Colony, Rly Qr. no. 530/4
P.O & Dist - Bilaspur (M.P.)
Pin - 495004

आपका
S.K.Vidyarthi

मुझे पूरा विश्वास है इसी विश्वास के तहत मैं आपको पत्र लिख रहा हूँ पत्रोत्तर शीघ्र देने की कृपा करियेगा मेरे पास समय का अभाव है मैं प्रतिदिन प्रतिपल आपके पत्र का ही इन्तजार करूंगा। पत्र yes or No में पूर्ण गोपनीयता के साथ अपने पास 20lhi में पहुंचे का इंतजाम जरूर भेजियेगा। गोपनीयता इसलिए जरूरी है कि कहीं हमारी कुर्बानी की भनक किसी को लग गयी तो मैं इसका दुष्परिणाम भुगतना पड़ सकता है। मैं 34 वर्षीय एक स्वस्थ 6 फिट लम्बा व्यक्ति हूँ मेरा वजन 88 kg. है मैं अपना एक, गुर्दा बेचना चाहता हूँ कृपया किसी पैसे वाले जरूरत मन्द से सौदा करवा दें। आप के पास लोगों लोग आते रहते है। P.T.O.

कार्बोर्ड

अथवा Contract, इसके अलावा मेरे पास
और कोई रास्ता नहीं है
Please sir मेरी बातों को गहराई से समझने
की कोशिश कीजिएगा।
४ आपके इन्तजार में,
शान्तनु कुमार
c/o छोटेलाल नाई की दुकान
आगरा मशीन के सामने
शिव नगर कालोनी
रायबरेली रोड़
फैजाबाद
यह पत्र में भावुकता में नहीं महीनों सोचने
समझने के बाद आपको लिख रहा हूँ।
पत्र श्रीपुत्ति श्रीघ्र व रजिस्टर्ड भेजन।
की कृपा करिएगा

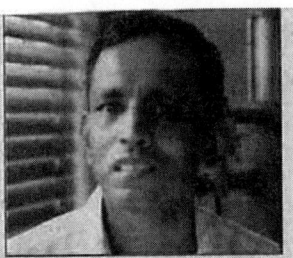

"None of my relatives' kidneys were suitable so I had to purchase one."
DR RAMACHANDRA RAO
Surgeon and renal patient

scrupulous middlemen. Bombay Hospital and the Guest Hospital in Madras are now directly advertising for donors, making payments for the kidneys themselves and ensuring after-care for the donors. A new phrase has even been coined called "rewarded gifting" to make it

MAXIMUM
CITY MUMBAI
KIDNEY TRADE
EPICENTRE

ATTEMPT TO LEGISLATE

Having realised the potential of such transplants an attempt was made to formulate and legislate the use of cadaver kidneys for the first time in India in the State of Maharashtra to which Bombay/Mumbai belongs. This law was called the 'Maharashtra Kidney Transplantation Act of 1982'. It was enacted by the Maharashtra Assembly in December 1982.

However, it became impossible to implement the same in view of the absence of 'Brain Stem death' criteria in this law. This needed a specific set of rules to be made for the purpose.

Meanwhile, as the problem of inadequate availability of donors from amongst the family members was mounting, some clinicians started using kidneys from 'unrelated' donors for transplants. Doctors Thiagarajan and Reddy reported their experience of more than thousand cases done by them by 1994, with some measure of success.[2]

However, in the impoverished developing world, this has led to commerce and trafficking in human organs with 'market forces' taking over with resultant trading in human organs, reports VN Acharya.

The 1982 Maharashtra Kidney Act for cadaver transplantation had no jurisdiction on the trade of kidneys from 'live donors' and so the lucrative enterprise by donors and their agents continued unabated.

---

[2] http://www.jpgmonline.com/article.asp?issn=0022-3859;year=1994; volume=40;issue=3;spage=158;epage=61;aulast=Acharya

Feeble attempts at making a difference by the Maharashtra Medical Council and Life Foundation were largely ineffective.

So dangerous was the game that makeshift transplant centres sprouted in converted apartments where patients were exposed to life-threatening infections.

Many West Asian patients – who underwent living unrelated kidney transplants in India – returned to their countries with bacterial and viral infections. *There was a high mortality rate among recipients and donors* with inadequate care, and commercial interest was paramount from beginning to end. The average cost of kidney and medical services in the 1990s was about ₹1.75 lakh. About ₹40,000 to ₹50,000 was paid to the donors who came from the slums and footpaths of Mumbai, the commercial capital of India. There were reports of missing persons who were kidnapped, and their kidneys removed to earn huge money.

At this juncture, strong opinions were expressed regarding the legal aspects of this unholy kidney bazaar in Mumbai. At that time, a senior advocate had been reported to have said, 'if my own relative needs treatment, I will not open the Indian Penal Code to examine the legality but open my wallet and save the patient (Indian Express, 8.7.1989)'.

Thus, Suketu Mehta's Maximum City acquired the dubious distinction of being the easiest and cheapest market for kidney trade, which continued to hold this status for many years.

Media started focusing on Mumbai in the late eighties. Rich Indians took their kidney donors from

MAXIMUM CITY MUMBAI KIDNEY TRADE EPICENTRE

the slums of Mumbai to London for a transplantation and the donor was allegedly paid between 2000 to 4000 pounds. As this became known, the print media worked over-time in England to highlight this exploitative practice by patients who took organs from the impoverished of Mumbai.

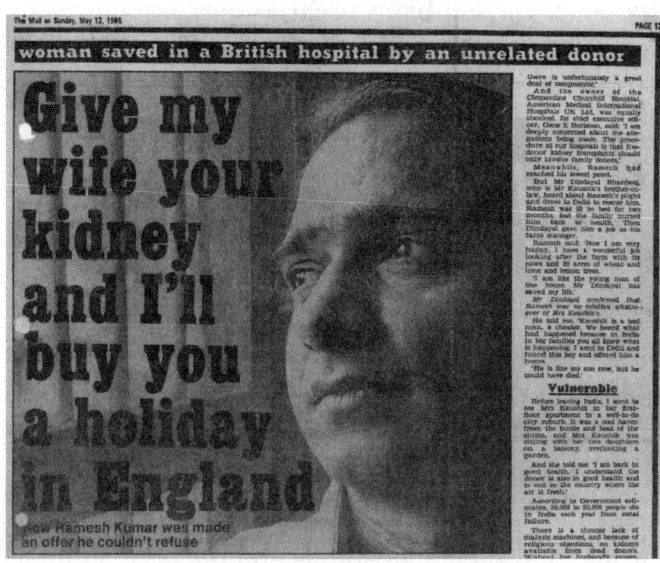

The Mail, 20 February 1985.

The nexus of surgeons, nephrologists and agents of private hospitals made large amounts of money at the expense of the poor through these unethical and gruesome practices. Unrelated transplantation in lesser-known hospitals of London such as Devonshire Hospital and Wessex Hospital occurred, sparking controversy when well-known surgeons participated for 'Blood Money' where poor donors were flown in from Bombay to London.

A prominent surgeon in London had at that time said, 'The transaction does not particularly bother me. If one person wishes to give another his kidney, I am prepared to take him as donor, as long as he understands what he is letting himself in for'.

The 'scandal of the wealthy' flourished with handsome dividends for surgeons and pittance to the poor. In Bombay's great kidney bazaar, well-protected networks between middlemen (*dalal*), laboratories, surgeons and nursing homes/hospitals were in place and a kidney transplant was possible within a week or so.

To make matters worse, the medical fraternity made statements in favour of buying kidneys for transplantation, and the print media highlighted such statement without any sense of responsibility on both sides. The practice was so rampant that by the '90s, nearly 100 transplants per month were being done in Bombay alone with a billion rupee/year industry in India. The real beneficiaries were the doctors, agents, hospitals and the poor, gullible donors were left behind.

Bombay's kidney bazaar: Thriving on donors' poverty States

Human organs for settling bank dues?

Hindustan Times, 9 February 1995.

MAXIMUM CITY MUMBAI KIDNEY TRADE EPICENTRE

Mumbai has the largest number of kidney transplant centres in the country today, including the more known Kokilaben Dhirubhai Ambani

Hospital, Jaslok Hospital, SL Raheja Hospital, Lilawati Hospital, Breach Candy Hospital, Fortis Hiranandani Hospital, Apollo Hospital, Nanavati Hospital, Fortis Hospital, Bombay Hospital, Bhatia Hospital, BYL Nair Charitable Hospital, Global Hospital, Godrej Memorial Hospital, KEM Hospital, Kohinoor Hospital, PD Hinduja Hospital and many others.

IN MORE RECENT TIMES

In 2015, an illegal kidney transplant racket came to surface at the Hiranandani Hospital in Powai area of Mumbai and it was alleged that a series of illegal transplants had been performed at this hospital.

In this case, the identity of a donor was changed to one Rashila Ben and her husband's to Bharat Bhai, and a deal of ₹3 lakh was struck with the husband for Rashila's kidney by a middleman alias Sandip, whose real name was said to be Brijendra Bisen. The surgery was done on 2nd May and follow-up and aftercare for both donor and recipient were forgotten.

The following year, another kidney racket was unearthed when on 14 July 2016 in the lobby of the Hiranandani Hospital, a social activist and Bahujan Samaj Party leader began frantically shouting about an illegal kidney transplant, flailing documents in the air until a police team arrived.

In this case, a 48-year-old sari-merchant from Surat was to undergo a kidney transplant from a donor who had migrated from Uttar Pradesh and declared that s/he was working as a domestic help, struggling to support five children. This deal was brokered by the same 'Bharat Bhai' whose wife 'Rashila Ben' had her kidney sold in the same hospital in 2015.

The CEO, medical director, nephrologist and two urologists were questioned, arrested and were let out on bail by the lower court. The transplant license of this hospital was canceled for a month. The police had arrested the transplant coordinator who was working as a link in this racket and a middleman for making forged documents; ₹8 lakh in cash was recovered from the residence of the transplant coordinator.

Two years after the organ transplant racket exploded in Hiranandani Hospital, a scam was busted in October 2018 in the famous JJ Hospital, one of the largest State-run hospitals in Maharashtra.

The State Anti-corruption Bureau had arrested two transplant coordinators for demanding a sum of ₹5 lakh from a Malad man awaiting clearance and approval for kidney transplant at the Raheja Hospital. Both were caught red-handed and arrested when they approached the patient's relatives to claim a part payment of ₹80,000.

As per Maharashtra government guidelines, organ transplants in the State including those conducted at private hospitals must be cleared by the JJ Hospital's Transplant Committee. Thus, Raheja and JJ, two hospitals were involved.

In 2018, the Anti-corruption Bureau of Maharashtra conducted a thorough scrutiny of 550 organ transplant cases, forwarded to the Transplant Authorisation Committee at the JJ Hospital by two apprehended transplant coordinators of JJ Hospital and Raheja Hospital since 2017. It was reported that a total of 32 kidney transplant cases were performed illegally through this nexus.

The State Health Ministry constituted a committee to investigate this kidney racket and the license of JJ Hospital itself to conduct further transplants was suspended until this enquiry was over.[3]

As a result, a new State Authorisation Committee was constituted and made responsible for investigating and authorising all applications for organ transplants in cases where a donor and a recipient were either distant relatives or unrelated.

---

[3] References: *The Times of India* 16.7.16, *The Indian Express* 17.7.16, *The Indian Express* 10.8.16, *The Pioneer* 11.8.16, *The Indian Express* 22.8.16, *Mumbai Mirror* 2.10.18, *Hindustan Times* 5.10.18.

KIDNEY RACKET IN TAMIL NADU

THE KIDNEY TRANSPLANTATION SCENE IN Chennai during the late 20th century was gruesome in terms of the exploitation of the impoverished.

This was coupled with the rampant practice of illegal transplantation at different nursing homes and hospitals, both registered and unregistered.

The Apollo Hospital, Chennai and Christian Medical College, Vellore had performed transplants where the patient had purchased the kidneys and a middleman was always involved. This practice was well established and led to the development of a semi-slum colony called Villivakkam on the outskirts of Chennai. The residents were extremely poor and at least one member of each family had sold his kidney, media reports said. The suburb was referred to as 'Kidneyvakkam' (*India Today*, 31 July 1990). This 'kidney colony' became so notorious in the international market that patients from neighbouring countries like Singapore and Thailand also lined up at Chennai to buy a 'live kidney'.

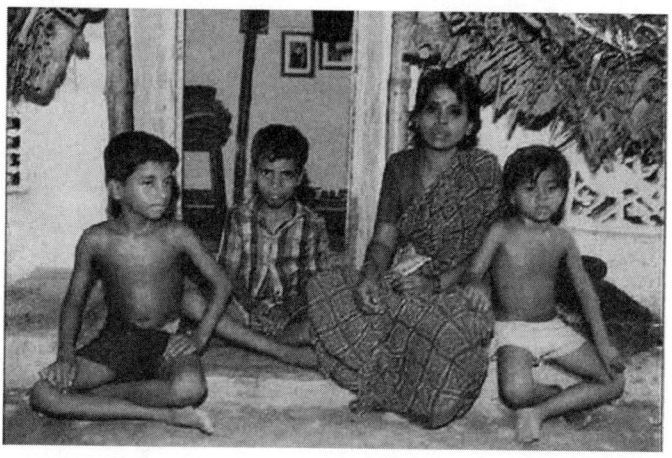

A media report said: Lakshmi Natarajan, 28, a mother of three, sold her kidney seven months ago for ₹25,000 and bought a house with the money. Her husband, an odd-job worker, had sold his kidney the year before to raise money for an auto-rickshaw.

Tamil Nadu had the attention of the world and it was a nightmare for all involved in this open, unethical practice of human exploitation.

In Chennai, the trade was open – where both male and female family members had sold their kidneys under the pressure of poverty and debt. Patients from all over the country formed a beeline to Chennai to buy a kidney from these poor people and returned to their homes after successful transplantation. The impact of poverty was so severe that donors were available in a queue at transplant centres in Chennai, Madurai and even in Vellore.

In the absence of proper legislation in the country, at the beginning, often contact between sellers and buyers occurred without the interference of middlemen. There were advertisements in national newspapers from patients in need of kidneys, and from those trying to sell their kidneys.

There was no restriction and very soon local middlemen and mafia took control of the procuring process and finding kidneys at the lowest possible price for the highest bidders. (*Transplantation Proceedings*, Vol 22, No.3 June 1990: pp 910–911) Transplantation took only a few years to become large-scale scams.

Although doctors across Chennai had agreed that it was unethical to allow the trading of human organs, they also asked whether it was ethical to let a patient die just because a blood-related donor could not be located. Senior nephrologists and surgeons in Chennai, Madurai and Vellore questioned the whole practice of 'unrelated kidney transplantation' and initiated a practice of a 'reward-gifting' in which the hospital took control of accepting and selecting a donor so that no middleman was engaged.

Estimates said that earlier about 140 transplants were performed in Chennai, and the recipients were from across India and also neighbouring countries. Once the reward-gifting scheme was put in place, the donor compensation was based upon socio-economic status, and the fee was collected by the hospital from the recipient. Nearly 300 to 400 such unconventional kidney transplantations from 'unrelated sources' were performed in Tamil Nadu hospitals in this period.

However, this model of unrelated kidney transplantation was not accepted across the nation and received criticism from the global community as well. The practice was also a stumbling block for cadaver transplantation in the country, since the impoverished were eager to receive money from any source, including kidney donation, either through middlemen or a hospital facility. It did not matter who gave the cash.

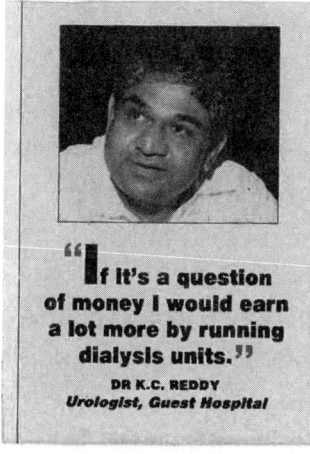

"If it's a question of money I would earn a lot more by running dialysis units."
DR K.C. REDDY
Urologist, Guest Hospital

And urologist Dr K.C. Reddy, whose Guest Hospital programme is among the better-run live unrelated donor programmes in the country, says: "If it's a question of money I would make a lot more running dialysis units. I'm not purchasing a kidney. I'm giving someone the gift of life. Tell me, what's so ethically objectionable about that?"

While most doctors acknowledge there are pressing needs for organ transplants they are not convinced by arguments to allow live unrelated donor transplants. They fear that it can never be regulated effectively and would go out of hand leading to exploitation and death. Says Dr M.K. Mani of Apollo Hospital: "Even with the best of intentions you can't police such a system and prevent the donor from being exploited. Secondly, we must build public opinion
K.V. ANAND

The kidney scams in Tamil Nadu had ramifications in Maharashtra, Gujarat, Karnataka and Kerala. Historically, Tamil Nadu had been a prominent centre for the treatment of kidney diseases – first at CMC Vellore and later the practice made progress in both government and private hospitals in the city of Chennai.

SCAMS INCREASE WITH DESTITUTION

In October 2007, a kidney racket was unearthed at St Thomas Hospital in Chennai where it was alleged that a practicing doctor was involved and he and his associates were booked under the THOA and Indian Penal Code (IPC).

Reports said, the surgical procedures were done in Bharti Raza Hospital and at St Thomas Hospital in Chennai and according to estimates, a total of 471 kidney transplants were done in these two hospitals in Chennai in the previous six years, with transactions worth around ₹100 crore.

This particular scam had country-wide ramifications. Media reports said, a gang assigned a middleman for each State of the country – to find prospective donors. These prospective donors were then taken to Palej town in Bharuch district of Gujarat, where the notorious agent Brijendra Bisen alias Sandip carried out extensive medical tests.

The donors were then brought to Tamil Nadu and kept in bungalows and farmhouses in Chennai, in allotted accommodations. In this whole racket, there was a bounty of ₹20 lakh per transplant. Out of this sum, ₹2 lakh was paid to an attorney for preparing the false documents needed for transplantation after 1994. Just ₹1 lakh was paid to the agent who had found the donor and brought him to Chennai. The donor was paid the least. The remaining amount was pocketed by the gang who operated the scam.

This scam ran for more than a decade. It was exposed when a daily-wage worker complained to unit-3 of the Mumbai Crime Branch that he was paid only ₹25,000 against the promised sum of ₹4 lakh for selling his kidney in Chennai.

In December 2004, hordes of people in Chennai became homeless and there was a sudden increase in kidney scams.

People had lost their homes, dwellings and livelihoods after a devastating tsunami struck the Tamil Nadu coastline. India was one of the 11 countries affected. People who had lost their homes and livelihoods had little hesitation in selling a kidney to make ends meet.

05 NOVEMBER 2007 | NATIONAL | CHENNAI KIDNEY TRADE

An Organ For A Dime

A Chennai doc's arrest shows the kidney trade continues to flourish in the city

Doctor Kingpin
- Conducted 471 kidney transplants in two Chennai hospitals in the last six years
- Charges Rs 15-Rs 20 lakh per operation. Is said to be worth Rs 100 crore. Owns three bungalows and three farmhouses in and around the city.
- Donors, most of them poor, gullible women, were lured by lakhs but paid only a few thousands

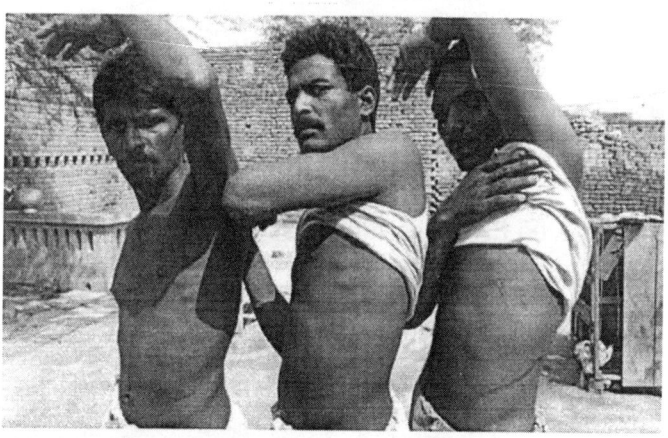

Cash for Kidneys: The 'Industry' That Preys on the Desperate - The Quint

In a scheme of selecting donors from poor families, females are preferred to their husbands who were mostly alcoholics and drug addicts.

With the connivance of a Chennai doctor – who was working 'hand-in-glove' with his counterpart in Sri Lanka – donors were flown to a few selected hospitals for transplantation in Sri Lanka. This particular channel of illegal kidney trade across and beyond the country came to surface when a donor – who needed money for her husband's plastic surgery – was simply paid ₹63,000, a sari and a supposedly gold bracelet.

Instead of husband's surgery, the woman used the money to pay her debts. She was sent to Sri Lanka with a false Indian passport and her name changed from Uma Devi to Govindamma in April 2005. A month later, she returned to India as Uma on a Sri Lankan passport.

This was an ingenious modality of using different country passports, adopted by the racketeers.[1] Using this method, kidney donors and recipients were freely travelling between Chennai and Sri Lankan hospitals. The lid came off when Uma was caught. Investigating teams in Chennai, Mumbai, Bengaluru, Hyderabad across India and in Sri Lanka began cooperating with each other to unearth the depth and dimensions of this international kidney scam. The outcome of this coordinated investigation, as usual, is not known.

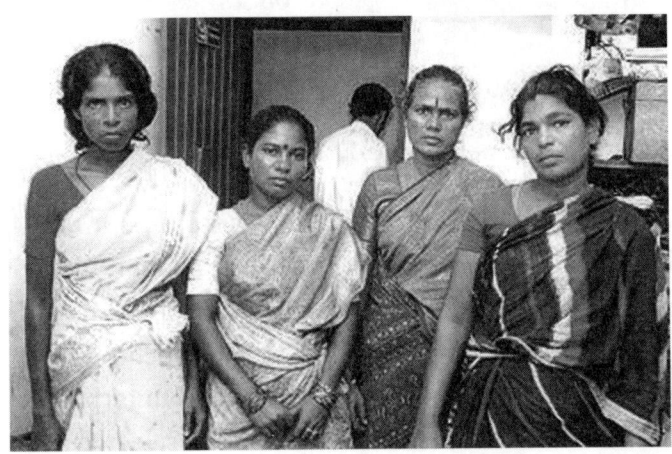

All these women have told the media that they had sold their kidneys.

[1] References: *The Indian Express* – 23.8.17, www.dnaindia.com – 10.10.07, www.outlookindia.com – 5.11.07, timesofindia.indiantimes.com – 22.6.16.

Chennai had by then earned a reputation of being a 'frontrunner' – both in organ donation and transplantation for kidneys and livers. Dr Sunil Shroff, Urologist and managing trustee of the Mohan Foundation (Multi Organ Harvesting Aid Network) had been a prominent component of transplant facilities in Chennai. According to the Transplant Authority of Tamil Nadu, a total of 5,385 transplants had been done in the city since 2008. The success rate of transplants was impressive and patients from across the country and neighbouring countries preferred to have their surgery done in Chennai.

The term 'medical-tourism' was coined here and used in the mainstream. But the clandestine activity of exploitative illegal transplantation has continued till date.

In India, during harvest seasons too, the buying and selling of kidneys as commodities increase as farming communities face cash crunch.

Recently, in a shocking development in Tamil Nadu, an organ transplant racket surfaced in 2018 where officials of the Union Ministry of Health and Family Welfare revealed that at least three hearts retrieved from brain-dead patients were given to international patients in Chennai.

There are strict guidelines for allocation of harvested organs under the direct control of National Organ & Tissue Transplant Organisation (NOTTO). They prescribe that an organ will be first offered to an Indian, or to a non-resident Indian (NRI), and an international patient can only be considered when neither are available. Organ trade, including heart and kidney trade, goes on in the garb of cadaver transplantation in India, despite the laws and numerous watchdogs.[2]

[2] Sep 10, 2018 | https://www.thehindu.com/news

BLOOD DONORS, DRUG MAFIA, DOWRY KIDNEYS IN KOLKATA

IN THE EIGHTIES, A WELL-STRUCTURED patient service of transplantation from related donors was prevalent in a few hospitals in Calcutta. The doctors working in these private hospitals teamed up with a breed of professional blood donors to create a living organs bank.

However, as elsewhere in the country, a gradual shift from related to unrelated donors began in these hospitals by the late eighties and to maintain high figures of transplants, an increasing number of 'cousins' began to be accepted.

Since some government hospitals were offering dialysis facilities free of cost, such as SSKM Hospital, it became a favoured place for patients, and soon it was unable to accommodate everyone; only patients with 'related' donors for transplantation were accepted for dialysis support. This resulted in the impersonation of donors, and in the absence of any prescribed guidelines to screen the donors, the practice of illegal transplantation continued unabated.

It is at this point that disappointed patients who were refused free hemodialysis and had no 'related' donors became prey to unscrupulous agents walking around dialysis units, in the corridors of hospitals. Each tout had created a nexus with hospital staff or doctors to obtain blood groups, financial status and residential status of such dialysis patients. A data bank of professional blood donors was accumulated from various blood bank centres with their meticulous records. With active participation and connivance of laboratories, the HLA profiles were readily available and matched to some extent with a prospective recipient.

The kidney-traders were clever enough to arrange meetings with the families of the recipient and the professional blood donor, only after large sums of money had been extracted from the recipient. The quantum of money transaction varied depending upon the desperation, eagerness and financial status of the recipient. The transactions varied between ₹80,000 to ₹1 lakh. The tout would take a lion's share of the money received and always warned the recipient's family to not disclose the quantum of transaction.

At this stage, the professional donor signed a declaration in the form of an affidavit that the kidney donation was on a voluntary basis. This documentation was necessary because common law does not allow a surgeon to remove an organ without voluntary consent and to prevent a criminal offence under section 126 of the IPC. Such a declaration was always by coercion, as all donors were extremely poor and in dire need of money, for purposes like alcohol addiction, re-payment of loans and dowry expenses of their daughter's marriages. It also included false promises of jobs etc.

In the early eighties, doctors in two Kolkata nursing homes were known to accept unrelated donors with affidavits from the courts endorsing 'close relationship with the recipient' and thus escaped any legal complications. In spite of knowing the details of the fraud, the transplants were carried out by doctors with personal benefits of ₹40,000 to ₹50,000 per case. A leading urologist and transplant surgeon, Dr Mohan Sil, who did most of the transplants at the Belle Vue Nursing Home, notably said: 'Although grafting an organ from an unrelated donor is unethical, how can I let a patient die if his relatives are unwilling to donate their kidney?' However, he expressed himself against the commercialisation of organs and said at that time that he kept being approached by middlemen willing to procure a kidney for his patients for a brokerage.

With well-established doctors' and middlemen nexus, the trade in Kolkata flourished with ever increasing queues of recipients seeking transplantation. Donors were chosen from the illiterate, malnourished, and drug-addicted professional blood donors. This was a gruesome practice, exploiting human beings with no ethics, morality and human values.

BLOOD DONORS, DRUG MAFIA

By the beginning of the 1990s, it was estimated that the kidney transplant trade had become a ₹6 crore industry in Kolkata. There was a lot of money involved in this business in the 1980s. The big players in this unholy work were kidney brokers, doctors, laboratories and to some extent, hospitals. This unethical business thrived as there was no law to check the kidney merchants. Donors were touted from the city slums or were professional blood donors in dire need of money. As for the prospective recipient, spending a few lakh rupees was within the reach of many needing transplantation, even if a suitable related sibling was available in the family for transplantation – a kidney purchased from the kidney bazaar was preferred.

Among the local population, there was always an apprehension to donate a kidney among the related family donors as kidney functions were perhaps better known. Parents here vehemently rejected organ donation from their grown-up children, then and even today. For financially stable recipients, it was not a problem to purchase a kidney. But for a poor recipient, it was an ongoing problem to incur monthly expenditure on dialysis amounting to thousands of rupees every month for their lifetime. In such a scenario, touts were always on the lookout, hanging around all dialysis facilities in the city. A typical case would play out thus:

A tout would make contact with the relatives of dialysis patients and offer services to arrange a kidney for transplantation. After a couple of meetings in the hospital, cafes and even at homes of such patients, depending upon the status and standard of living, a tout would enhance the quantum of the deal. Of course, the entire proceedings of these transactions were done in secrecy and a nexus of doctors, middlemen, nursing homes, diagnostic centres and laboratories inside and outside the hospital were firmly in place for recipients seeking transplantation.

In Kolkata, however, gradually the easy availability of professional blood donors dried up, as donating blood two or three times a week would fetch only ₹20 to ₹30 per donation, and such small money would end up in country liquor dens. Earning a large amount of ₹25,000 to ₹50,000 for a kidney was more attractive. In this situation, even blood banks started arranging kidneys for sale, and the brokerage and detection of this transaction was nearly impossible in the absence of any receipt issued.

This unethical practice developed channels of luring patients for transplantation from abroad, such as Singapore and middle eastern countries and soon India became an international kidney bazaar where one could shop around for a decent kidney at the best price. Kidney merchants took advantage of the lack of laws to check this trade of exploitation of the poor. All others involved in a transplant except for the donor victims, earned big amounts of money with impunity. The recipient actually bought the gift of life.

After the Transplantation Act came in force in 1994–1995, the open illegal kidney transplant activity slowed down, but reports from the sector say, it has continued underground for the last 25 years with equal zeal and still continues, governments unable to stop the trade.

In November 2017, four people were arrested for active involvement in a kidney transplant racket in a private hospital in Kolkata. The documents recovered from the arrested proved that the racket in kidneys continues. The identity of the accused, the kingpin, his wife with their associates also became known. Heroin weighing 316gm, with a market value of ₹3 lakh, was also seized from those arrested. This added a new dimension to the crime and money earned from exploiting the poor. For the first time, the drug angle to this narrative became visible.

Another recent case was that of a young woman in Kolkata. The practice of dowry – getting paid to marry a girl and gifted as demanded – was banned in India in 1961 and stronger laws were introduced in 1980 to protect married women from cruelty. This particular case received the attention of foreign media, the *Telegraph* and the *Washington Post*.

Following her marriage in 2005, this woman was under constant pressure from her husband and his family for a dowry. In 2016, about ten years after her marriage, she was admitted to a private medical facility for appendectomy. As her pain continued, her father took her to another facility where an ultrasound showed her kidney had been taken illegally.

The police arrested the woman's husband and his brother from Murshidabad district near Kolkata. The husband then confessed that he and his brother had sold the woman's kidney to a businessman in Chhattisgarh.

In July 2018, in a northern suburb of Kolkata, an accused escaped arrest due to a tipoff from a woman who was seeking a kidney donor in south Kolkata. He took the contract for the supply of kidneys for the price of ₹5 lakh. The money was collected and concealed in fruit-baskets during the period of admission in the nursing home for transplantation.

The malpractice of kidney transplantation from unrelated paid donors continues in Kolkata even as we write, and a couple of my patients have paid hefty amounts of money to find a kidney donor and get transplant surgery done in the city. I was very surprised and very curious as to know what happened to see them on their return from Kolkata. This got me thinking.

Recently, the Naihati police in the North 24 Parganas district of Kolkata apprehended nine people in a kidney supply network. The mastermind of the racket is still untraceable. Their network is believed to be spread from Bihar, Jharkhand, Assam, Uttarakhand to Rajasthan, and the investigation has so far led to a 'fake document racket' conducted from a shop in Natun Bazar, Jalpaiguri. This is just the tip of the iceberg of a very well-organised scam network that exists in the region.[1]

---

[1] References: *The Washington Post*, 9th February 2018; www.indianexpress.com, 3rd July 2018 ; *The Indian Express* – 10.9.18.

THE KIDNEY KING AND THE GREAT ESCAPE

THE GURUGRAM KIDNEY SCANDAL IS a multi-billion-rupee racket which had ramifications on a national and international scale, led by an untrained non-medical and self-proclaimed 'surgeon'. For the purpose of our story, let us call him K – the Kingpin of the racket in Gurugram, close to Delhi.

The donors were impoverished victims, in recent years, mostly hailing from nearby western Uttar Pradesh. This horrific self-claimed surgeon, an Ayurveda practitioner, carried out 600 illegal kidney transplants between 1996 to 2008.

K's younger brother L, who was his assistant in this crime, moved from one city to another, got arrested several times and obtained quick bail. The kingpin had a very close and strict relationship with his younger brother, who was overall in-charge of the venue of their activities, and the payments received were in crores, Sumitra, the brother's wife told investigators.

The kingpin's son M, from his first marriage, a 35-year-old and also involved in his racket, is still absconding. This family run a mafia and operate on an international scale.

There is no fixed rate charged for the transplantations this gang performs and the charges vary from ₹10 lakh to ₹60 lakh, depending on the *richness* of the recipient. The clients are from the United States of America, the United Kingdom, Canada, Saudi Arabia, Greece, Oman, Israel, Russia, as well as many wealthy Indian citizens. The poor donors whose kidneys are removed, however, are paid only between a few thousand rupees to a lakh per case.

The gang has performed illegal transplants in Jaipur, Gurugram, Faridabad, Ambala, Panchkula in Haryana, Guntur in Andhra Pradesh, and Anand in Gujarat. *It is inconceivable but true that they obtained bail each time a member was apprehended by the police in every city, which only demonstrates the reach of their money and power.* The kingpin changed his name in each place to facilitate his illegal activity in each city.

According to media reports, this gang K's transplantation activities started in the early nineties in Mumbai at the Kaushalya Nursing Home, Khar where K had invited several renal surgeons and doctors from other hospitals, well-known in the city (as per a statement by the wife of the kingpin's brother). In Mumbai, K had taken the help of good-looking nurses who would persuade donors. The donors were mainly labourers, taxi drivers and beggars. Many of these donors were found while hanging around Mahim and Haji Ali Dargah and the city temples.

A few underpaid labourers approached the police and filed a complaint which is what led to K's first arrest in 1995 in Mumbai. *However, K was influential, and he managed to obtain bail immediately.* He was in police custody just for a month before he obtained bail.

From Mumbai, he had setup a base in Vapi and then in Nepal under the patronage of a Member of Parliament. The chief investigator in the Mumbai case said that this 'doctor' was a 'professional cheat' who would go to any extent for money, and his clients were rich Arabs.

By 1995, there was an organ transplant law in the country, but not strong enough to deter K. He obtained bail each time and shifted his operation to Jaipur, Guntur and Hyderabad.

In another case filed against him in May 2005, on the charges of duping a local individual, *K was released after police failed to file the chargesheet in the stipulated time of 90 days*. In this case, the complainant was brought to Gurgaon, in the NCR region, underwent kidney removal for a promised amount of ₹3 lakh but was ultimately paid only ₹70,000.

By this time, the police and media had a lot of information on K, but neither acted on the available information. The police and media, and the authorities knew that the kingpin was also planning to open his own hospital in various parts of the country. One such hospital was in Sadhopur village of Noida, where the construction was stopped following K's arrest.

Ironically, K was granted bail in several other criminal cases pending against him while he was serving his sentence in Ambala Jail.

The kingpin of this operation, K, was born 65 years ago. He has two brothers, the other two now of the ages 55 and 50 years respectively and both closely linked to his kidney racket. They were natives of Akola in Maharashtra.

A MAN WITH GREAT ACTING SKILLS

The eldest of the siblings, K was an ayurvedic practitioner and all three brothers initially worked together at their Mumbai clinic in the 1990s. During this time the kingpin worked under his birth name, but once he began getting involved in illegal activities and throughout the rest his career so far, he has operated under many different names and addresses. In the media he is known as Amit Kumar, one of his brother is called J Rao or Jeevan Kumar but if these are their real names – is not known.[1]

In Mumbai, K had a multifarious and colourful profile in the early nineties and funded C-grade films. K and his younger brother L, had also acted in a film called *Khooni Raat*, in which he played a cop. It was widely known that he had a keen interest in acting and acted in other B and C grade films such as *Kanoon Ki Janjeer* and *Aag*.

---

[1] https://www.hindustantimes.com/india-news/the-fallrise-and-fall-of-kidney-racket-kingpin-dr-amit-kumar/story-hgMheixL8H9l6k1KTNeNCN.html

While in Mumbai, he started a film company called 'Film World' which never took off. He married thrice, and his present wife is a former Miss Chandigarh, a 35-year-old with an MBA who worked at a bank until 2010. Even if he no longer acts, K's power to convince and dupe has only grown stronger and this is his biggest asset in his criminal activities. He can convince anyone – his wives, the authorities, the police and the courts, the recipients and donors, even members of India's hallowed Parliament.

K soon shifted his illegal activities from Mumbai to Gurugram (then 'Gurgaon', a part of the National Capital Region). The brothers set up a hospital in Gurugram – the Star Max Hospital, at House No.2374, Sector-23 registered in the name and style of M/s Liberty Health Care Limited. In the subsequent years, they set up several other hospital facilities in and around Delhi.

The kidney donors were poor and gullible individuals hunted by a team of touts operating in western Uttar Pradesh. The touts worked like professional headhunters, seeking all the eligibility details, personal profiles and matching all parameters to their programme's specific requirements. They had donor data at the tip of their fingers.

These donors were given as little as ₹5000 to ₹70,000 to sell their kidneys to this hospital. These were then sold at astronomical costs of ₹10 lakh or more taken from foreign recipients. The kingpin did not even spare his ward boy, who he convinced to part with one of his kidneys for just ₹10,000 when he could not find a donor for a rich client.

On 24 January 2008, after a labourer in Moradabad complained of harassment by cronies of this nefarious kidney kingpin, the Moradabad police and the Delhi/Haryana police teams raided the Star Hospital in a joint operation.

Amit Kumar alias K managed to abscond and at this point of time, the Moradabad police arrested his accomplice in surgery from a hotel in Faridabad, while the Gurugram police arrested four of their agents from the residence cum hospital in Gurugram. According to a first-person account, just a few minutes before the police raid the scene at the hospital was horrific:

> There were five donors admitted and on various beds in the hospital and their lives were in a pathetic condition. They were told that just a few minutes before, 'the doctor has been caught and the police is coming'. So, what the hospital staff did was remove all the donors' blood drips and glucose and said, 'You also run away from here'. Their kidneys were operated on that same day a few hours earlier, and the donors were just left like this and there was no one to take care of them and one of the patients was actually writhing in pain.

The following day, on 25 January, five foreign nationals – Joy Mehtal, 53 yrs and his wife Sonam Joy, 52 yrs, a US-based NRI couple; and three Greek citizens Leonida Dayasi, 56 yrs; Leonidas Dayasi, 63 yrs; and Heleni Kitcocy, 53yrs; were found awaiting kidney transplants in a guesthouse owned by the kingpin.

The police also rescued five Indian people from various parts of northern India, from another

Gurugram hospital – obviously they were prospective donors.

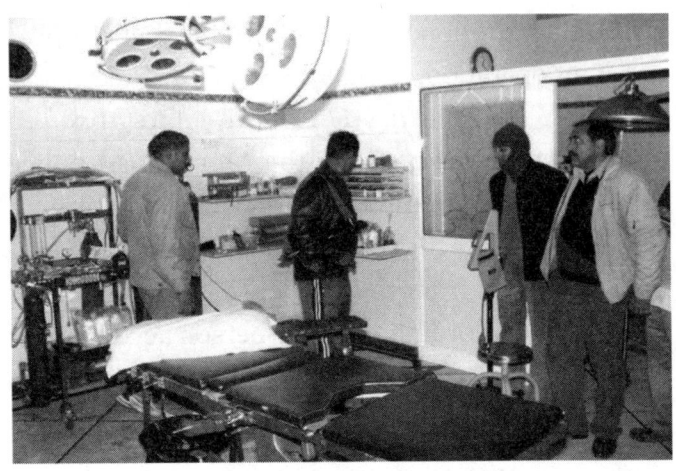

Haryana police raiding the illegal Gurugram transplant facility.

At that time, the Gurugram police chief said that the kingpin and his associates had been arrested thrice before for illegal organ transplants in Delhi, Andhra Pradesh and Maharashtra, and that they had fled after receiving bail each time. The police had also uncovered two more hospitals and ten laboratories in the National Capital Region (NCR) involved in this racket.

Eight luxury cars that ferried the patients were seized in addition to eight bank accounts. On 29 January, the then Union Health Minister, asked for a CBI[2] probe and an Interpol alert with a red-corner notice against the kingpin and his brother was

---

[2] India's prime investigating agency, the Central Bureau of Investigation.

initiated. The brother's wife and the kingpin's driver were arrested on the charges of criminal conspiracy.

K was finally arrested from a hotel in the holiday resort, Chitwan, 35 miles from the border between India and Nepal on 7th February 2008.

The hotel staff got suspicious of his behaviour because he was wearing a hat and sunglasses indoors and was noticed cutting out stories about the Indian kidney scam from local Nepali newspapers.

At the time of his arrest, he had a bank draft for ₹9 lakh and cash piles of €140,000 and $20,000 on him. After his arrest, he was taken to Kathmandu and paraded before journalists. Even at the resort, as soon as he was arrested, he made an unsuccessful attempt to bribe two Nepalese policemen to let him go.

Making a statement of his innocence, K averred on Nepali Television channel that, 'I have not committed any crime'. He said, he was attempting to flee to Canada where he owned a home. He had well-established connections in some private hospitals in Kathmandu such as Om Hospital, where there was suspicion of a kidney racket as well.

With intensive negotiations between the Police Commissioner of Kathmandu and the Director of the CBI in India, K was handed over to Indian authorities on 9 February 2008, with ₹1.22 crore recovered from him in foreign currency.

A criminal case against K and his gang members was registered on 8 February 2008 by the CBI under section 120-B, 326, 342, 417, 465, 473, 506 and 307 of IPC. It took the CBI four years to frame charges against ten of the gang members accused.

THE CASE OF THE SLEEPING POLICEMEN

On 22 March 2013, a special court held five persons guilty. In their order, the special CBI Judge at the Panchkula court awarded a seven-years jail sentence and imposed a fine of ₹60 lakh each on K and his brother L. Another three were sentenced for five years of rigorous imprisonment and a fine of ₹15,000 each. The remaining accused – including K's brother J Rao – and two other doctors and a nurse were acquitted.[3] The court also ordered a compensation of ₹10 lakh each for three victims – Shahid, Sakil and Babu Ram.

On the quantum of sentence, the CBI special judge said the convicts, being in the medical health sector, were associated with 'the most noble profession' and:

> Each and every human being reposes faith in the medical fraternity and the convicts have shaken that faith. Being doctors and those associated with medicine, they committed inexcusable sin in society while their responsibility was far greater than what one expects of a common man.

With this 2013 CBI sentence, K was lodged in the Ambala Jail in Haryana, outside the NCR.

In addition to this sentence, a Faridabad court, on 28 February 2012, had sentenced K and another

---

[3] https://zeenews.india.com/news/haryana/gurgaon-kidney-racket-kingpin-dr-amit-convicted_837210.html

man who also claimed to be a doctor, U Durgesh, to 10 years of rigorous imprisonment in connection with the death of three Turkish nationals – Mehmat Bijayat (2003), Ismat Gunnar (2004) and Ahmed Yeliders (2005). The two so-called doctors were held guilty for 'negligence' in their treatment of kidney transplantation and deaths that had come to light only after the kidney racket surfaced in 2008. It had taken seven years for these foreign patients to get some kind of retribution.

The Gurugram kingpin had another case pending against him after he had conducted surgeries – removing the kidneys – of thirteen victims from Pandoli village near Anand, Gujarat. A man called Aamir Malek, a villager, had filed a complaint with the Petlad police saying that his kidney had been extracted without his knowledge in a Delhi hospital.

K was brought to the Tees Hazari Court in New Delhi on 29 July 2016, where he was to appear for a hearing in connection with another similar kidney racket case. A team of three members of the Anand Crime Branch arrested him from Tees Hazari, on his arrival in court.

K was escorted from Delhi to Anand by the Gujarat police on the Swarna Jayanti Express on 9 August. On guard were one police inspector and two policemen. K was allegedly hand-cuffed to a railing in a train compartment. According to these policemen, all of them had dinner together. The police team went to sleep after that.

It was sometime between 2 a.m. and 3 a.m. when the train was crossing Ajmer Junction that one of the police constables woke up and found K, their important prisoner, missing from his seat. The handcuff was intact and still latched to the railing.[4]

Of course, the escape from police custody speaks of great negligence, which were both purposeful and paid-for heavily. After his August 2016 escape, K was declared an absconder and a reward of ₹50,000 was announced for information on him by the Gujarat Police.

K and his gang earned in crores and spending a few lakhs was not a big deal for him. *He was able to obtain bail from courts anywhere in the country and got away with hefty bribes at every step of his multiple arrest.*

STILL GOING STRONG

On 11 September 2017, the Uttarakhand police busted an illegal kidney racket at the Gangotri Charitable Hospital, situated 35 kilometers from Dehradun city.

Four days later, after a hectic search, the Gurugram kidney kingpin was arrested from Panchkula in Haryana, along with his brother, while his son escaped. Other individuals arrested were a staff nurse, a cook and a driver. As much as ₹33 lakh in cash were also found. It was alleged that 50 illegal transplants were conducted between July and September 2017 at that hospital outside Dehradun.

[4] https://timesofindia.indiatimes.com/city/vadodara/Kidney-doctor-flees-from-train-as-cops-dozedoff/articleshow/53625944.cms

K's third wife, a beauty queen who had married him in 2014, made a statement to the court that she was unaware of his whereabouts until his latest arrest in Dehradun in September 2017. She recalled having received cake and a bouquet of flowers on her birthday, but the place from where the bouquet was sent was not legible on the tag. Similarly, in 2013, when he was in jail in Guntur, Andhra Pradesh, she says she had met him on July 16 on his birthday and given him a cake. The wife had met him in the jail and claimed that she had been borrowing from relatives for her own expenses and pronounced that 'he is a good person' – unlike his brother J Rao (sic), she said.

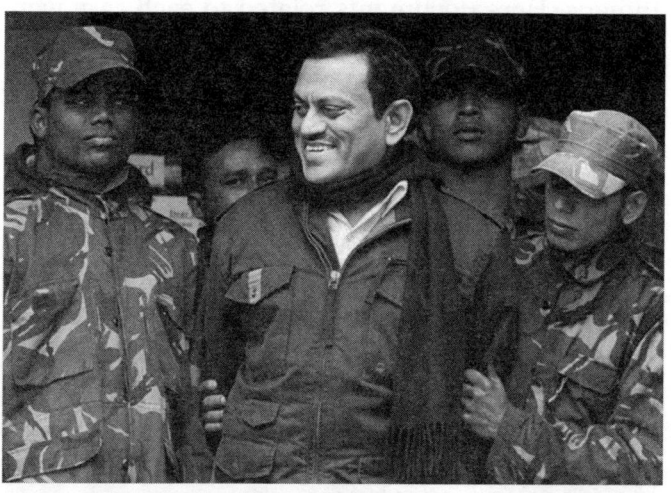

Media image of the kingpin of the Gurugram kidney racket, K, in police custody.

When the 'Gurgaon Kidney Scandal' was busted in 2008, this 'Dr Horror' had been arrested multiple times and had managed at most times to escape. But, with this latest arrest in late 2017, the kingpin's luck finally seemed to have run out.

K was unable to bribe the police constable from the Haridwar police on duty and his accomplices, natives of Mumbai, were arrested along with the owners of the hospital where the transplants were conducted.

It was discovered that a makeshift operation theater had been made in a building at a desolate location on the Dehradun-Haridwar highway, and post-operative cases were kept at Gangotri Charitable Hospital, situated in the compound of the Uttaranchal Dental College, Lal Tappad, Doiwala. The recipients were predominantly residents of Oman and wealthy Indians. Here documents related to each case were burned to eliminate any evidence and the recipients and donors were asked to leave after two to three days. The laboratory investigations were conducted in Delhi. In this racket, an Omani national's papers were seized in a car at Doiwala near Dehradun.

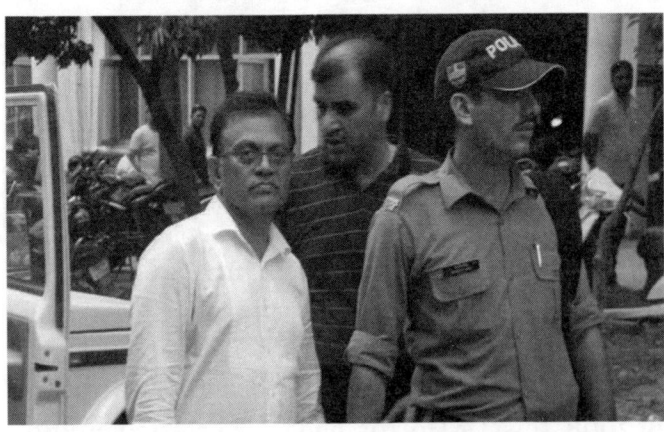

The kingpin in police custody.

K and his team would not have been able to carry on with their nefarious illegal kidney trade without a strong network of touts and middlemen who line up kidney donors and recipients from different parts of the country and abroad.

At present, K is lodged in Dehradun District Jail.

It is only a matter of time that he will be out of jail on bail, as he has done many many times in the past. This is the irony of law and the system as a whole in India – a man who has run a multi-nation illegal kidney racket for 20 years can soon be free to resurface somewhere else. The north or south, it matters not to him, as long as his donor supply continues. And this continues as poverty continues in India and the greed to make a quick buck operates in the open market and without any moral and ethical constraints.[5]

---

[5] References: https://timesofindia.indiatimes.com/city/delhi/kidney-racket-busted-in-Gurgaon;https://www.dailypioneer.com/state-editions/dehradun/kidney-scam-sit-team-inspects-room-of-accused.html;https://www.thehindu.com/todays-paper/tp-national-newdelhi/bail-granted;https://www.thehindu.com/todays-paper/IsquoKidney-racket-mastermind;https://timesofindia.indiatimes.com/city/gurgaon/Gurgaon-kidney-scam;https://www.mohanfoundation.org/news/indian-kidney-king-would-not-spare;https://indianexpress.com/article/india/surgery-racket-held-in-dehradun;https://indianexpress.com/article/cities/ahmedabad/kidney-racket-busted;https://www.hindustantimes.com/india-news/the-fall-rise-and-fall;

https://www.hindustantimes.com/dehradun/kidney-racket-dehradun-police Man who ran kidney rackets for 20 years held, yet again, Dehradun News – *The Times of India* – 17.9.17.

KIDNEY SCANDAL IN KARNATAKA

IN THE FIRST DECADE OF the new century, the medical world was shocked to read incredible reports appearing in the press about kidney transplant rackets in Bangalore hospitals going on for several years. It was reported that over 1,000 unrelated kidney removals were undertaken from underprivileged donors for paltry sums.

This kidney transplant racket in Karnataka was humongous in its depth and ramification and was considered at par with the racket in Mumbai. There was widespread publicity worldwide. Newspaper reports ran:

> The widespread racket came to surface when a coolie named Velu, a 29-year-old from Alamedu village in the Erode district in Tamil Nadu, was approached by a middleman for a job in Bangalore. This middleman, along with two other middlemen, kept Velu in a small hotel for a week. Velu was cajoled into donating blood for earning small sums of money. Agreeing to be a blood donor, the unsuspecting Velu underwent multiple tests and was

admitted to the Yellamma Dasappa Hospital, where he was examined by two doctors.

Velu was allegedly taken to an operation theatre to 'donate blood', and after the effect of anaesthesia had worn off, he was told that the big bandage in his abdomen was put for an injury sustained during a fall. Later, other villagers from the region also claimed that they too were duped of their kidneys through this process of 'blood donation'.

The police arrested two doctors: one senior nephrologist and one associate. The investigations concluded that the modus operandi was that the associate doctor would contact rich people in countries like Saudi Arabia, and once a rich patient was located, a poor villager would be brought to the hospital under the guise of giving blood on payment – but instead, a kidney was removed from the donor.

The police were able to detect 100 such cases in which kidneys were taken without consent and sold at astronomical prices. The villagers were paid a sum of a few thousand rupees. It is possible that some villagers may have given their kidneys willingly and once the scam erupted, they decided to come forward to testify. The police arrested four doctors, three middlemen, and the medical director of Yellamma Dasappa Hospital and the hospital's license was suspended for one year by the Karnataka Medical Council.

During that period, 2000–2010, it was estimated that, on the average, 300 transplants were carried out per year in Bangalore. The documents of other hospitals like the Mallya Hospital, Manipal Hospital,

MS Ramaiah Hospital and Lakeside Hospital were also reviewed by the authorities but unfortunately, the outcome of this scrutiny is not available in the public domain. For a doctor, especially a nephrologist, it is beyond imagination that 300 transplants were carried out in a couple of hospitals in a year in just one city – Bangalore and this practice was flourishing for 3 to 4 years.

Illegal donation of kidneys is widespread in Bangalore and executed with meticulous precision, through mutual cooperation. The police in this district raided a house on a tipoff, preventing five people from becoming victims of the kidney trade in 2007. The main accused and middlemen were practicing this illegal trade for seven years and had duped 25 kidney donors by August 2007.

His two accomplices – one, himself a kidney donor – authenticated the documents before a magistrate. Such documents were presented to the Authorisation Committee in Bangalore and from there it would be sent for police verification. Long before police inspection in the villages, the potential donors would be shifted to the same location as the recipients, so that the neighbours could vouch for the donors, after they were paid for their services, of course. The kidney recipients were tutored, and the Authorisation Committee would clear the application.

The donors were poor farmers and a couple were sick weavers, all under debt to money lenders. This racket came to light on complaints of a young man called Narasimha, who was searching for a money lender, and landed up in the clutches of the kidney racket middlemen.

Eventually, the two accomplices were also arrested.

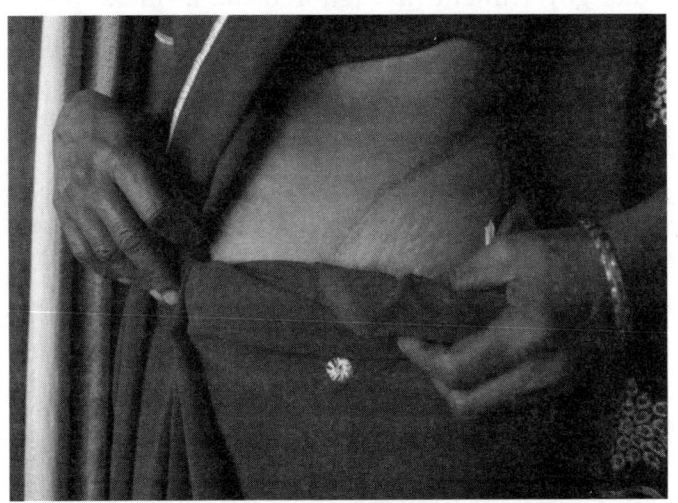

A woman donor detained in Bangalore kidney racket.
Source: *The Hindu*, 12 June 2016.

On 15 July 2015, another kidney racket came to light when a donor had a fight with the middleman over sharing of ₹10 lakh taken from the recipient. It is alleged that the donor was paid ₹3 lakh instead of the fifty per cent that was agreed upon. The recipient, middleman and donor were all booked.

Soon, a few other exploitation stories came to the notice of the police, as organ donation and selling had become a very common practice in that region of Karnataka. In the majority of cases, it is alleged that the donor was promised ₹10 lakh for donating a kidney and in the process, the middleman pocketed

KIDNEY SCANDAL IN KARNATAKA

as much as ₹6 lakh of that ₹10 lakh without informing the donor. Typically, the donors received ₹3–4 lakh in each transaction. As agricultural distress in the region grew, crop losses had continued, and the State government had ignored the farmers' plight repeatedly in those years. This is when the activities of the middlemen increased, and their illegal businesses flourished across Karnataka.[1]

[1] References: *The Hindu* – 13.8.07, India Today – 17.6.13, *Mail Online* – 21.7.15.

TRIBALS AS KIDNEY DONORS IN KERALA

IN MARCH 2018, THE CITY police of Kochi arrested a 50-year-old man (named Q) residing at Kumbalangi on the charges of forcing and intimidating a man called Dileep, a resident of Udayamperoor, for backing out of a deal to donate his kidney for ₹6 lakh.

This man, Q, was arrested from a nearby hospital at Panangad.

Allegedly, the complainant had received an advance of ₹15,000 for the donation of a kidney to a 12-year-old boy suffering from end stage kidney disease admitted in a private hospital in Kochi.

Further investigations had revealed that there was an organised kidney racket involving some private hospitals in the city, *but the local police said, it had no evidence to link management personnel of these hospitals to the kidney racket.* Q had told the police that a few hospital employees were also involved in identifying patients in need of kidney transplantation.

'God's own Country', Kerala, came under the police spotlight when *Madhyamam*, a Malayalam Daily, in 2002 published the story of an illegal kidney trade thriving in and around the Poomala-Maythotti tribal settlement in Idukki district.

In the first report, it was disclosed that 9 people, including 5 tribal people, were made to 'donate' their kidneys in previous years and payments had been made to them. Private hospitals in Kozhikode, Kochi and Thrissur were also involved in this scam.

TRIBALS AS KIDNEY DONORS IN KERALA

Unscrupulous racketeers tightened their grip on these tribes when the tribal people from the Ulladas, Ooralis, Aaryas communities and the 'Dalits' openly said that they survive by selling kidneys. The members of the kidney-selling gangs were quite astonished to see so many coming forward to sell kidneys for ₹1.5 lakh each, without any persuasion. Thus, Poomala began to be known as the 'Kidney Village' among middlemen.

On 10 June 2002, two men from the tribal settlement in Idukki alleged at a press conference at the press club at Kottayam that they were duped into selling their kidneys on the false promise of hefty compensation. They were escorted by the opposition, Kerala Congress members, and it was disclosed that a person called Mr 'R' was the kingpin and middleman in this scam.

The Left alliance was in power at the time in the State. The Chief Minister then ordered a police enquiry and asked for a report to be submitted within three months. The State Human Rights Commission and Scheduled Castes and Tribes Welfare Committee of the Kerala Assembly had initiated an inquiry of its own. The Kerala Branch of the Indian Medical Association had also constituted a three-member committee to enquire into the allegations. *Surprisingly, the IMA concluded that the donation of kidneys could not have taken place without the concurrence of the donors (sic).*

The State Minister for Scheduled Castes and Scheduled Tribe Development made a statement that the victims were 'not too poor and starving' as reported in the media. After an uproar in the media and the public against a doctor involved, who was a relative of the State Minister, in the scam, it was suggested that all regulations were followed in the kidney donation and donors had done so of their own free will.

The leader of opposition in the State assembly and a Congress team had visited the tribal colony in Idukki and had found that the report of illegal kidney trade was true and claimed that all the enquiries made by different agencies was a farce. They also indicted the Authorisation Committee for approving the cases and said the doctors at private hospitals in Kozhikode should face legal actions for conducting such operations.

The authorities of these private hospitals denied their involvement in a press conference and absolved themselves of participation in the kidney racket. The single Authorisation Committee based in Kozhikode was, however, dismissed, and three separate Authorisation Committees for the south, central and northern zone of the State were constituted for streamlining the transplant activities in the State.

TRIBALS AS KIDNEY DONORS IN KERALA

One 'KR' of neighbouring Kasipalayam had accompanied a gang of touts to a private hospital at Ernakulam in Kerala for selling one of his kidneys. His wife, working as a tailor in a garment manufacturing unit, was unaware of her husband's decision and had filed a complaint with the local police in Erode, Tamil Nadu.

Earlier, a kidney broker from Avinashi (Tirupur district) had convinced him of a large amount of money if he sold one of his kidneys. Based on the wife's complaint, a police team from Erode reached the VPS Lakeshore Hospital on time, and the transplant was stopped on the basis that his wife had not given any consent, which was necessary for transplantation. 'KR' was thus rescued and travelled back to Erode.

Bargain, Buy and Sell Kidneys

On the way back from Poomala Methotti after talking to the tribals who sold their kidneys, a call was made to the mobile phone number of the racket, given by the tribals.

"98472 62412"

-Hello who is it? A rough voice on the other side.

-Calling from Poomala. Calling after talking to Kunju who sold his kidney.

-We talked about O+ve kidney to Kunju.

-Yes I am unemployed'. Would like to sell O+ve kidney.

-Come to ………. hospital at Indira Gandhi Road, Kozhikode. You will be given one rupee.

-One?

-One Lakh. Are you married? How old are you?

-33, married.

-Did you talk to your wife?

> -No
>
> -Talk to her and come to Kozhikode today itself. If she is willing her kidney also will be taken. For that the money is 1.5 Lakhs. It is difficult to get kidneys of women. Everything should be in secret.
>
> -After coming to the hospital what should I do?
>
> -Call this number. – The phone went off.
>
> This is how the racket buys kidneys from Poomala Methotti. George was the first

An extract from PK Prakash's investigative reports on Kidney racket in Kerala (http://pkprakash.com).

The tribal kidney racket in Kerala consisted of money power, muscle power and political power. It also had components of deceit and duping of potential recipients and swindling lakhs of rupees on the false promise of finding a suitable kidney donor.

In 2014, the city police in Kochi arrested 'PPR' of Kanjiramkulam, Thiruvananthapuram, suspected to be the kingpin behind the scam.

The arrest was made on two complaints, one made by a student Ajay and another by a resident of Chathannoor in Kollam. It was reported in the local media that the kingpin himself underwent medical tests, and when his kidney did not match with the father of Ajay, a second donor was presented who was found suitable to donate.

In December 2012, the Authorisation Committee cleared the case. In transplant records, the paid donor was shown as a driver employed by the family and had offered his kidney 'out of love and affection' to the recipient. After the committee meeting, Ajay's father paid ₹3 lakh to 'PPR', the tout, and the approved kidney donor, and both men then vanished. The patient's relatives claimed that they had met 'PPR' through a newspaper advertisement for kidney donors that they had put out themselves. This whole episode happened in 2011, despite the Transplant Act that was already in place.

Soliciting kidney donors through print or visual media is prohibited by the Transplantation Act. But this case shows how people flout the law.

TRIBALS AS KIDNEY DONORS IN KERALA

Here was a case of 'double fault' where large sums of money were paid, and advertisements were given in newspapers. It only shows that the observance and practice under the strict guidelines of the Act were flouted by all. The newspapers know very well that such advertisements are prohibited. The general public too are aware that there are rules and regulations guiding organ donation because the laws themselves have been in place for 25 years. Missionaries, NGOs, educational institutions in these tribal areas too are aware of the rules. By placing an open ad for purchase, the recipient family is equally culpable. Then, of course, there is the donor, who, as the then government noted, was a voluntary donor, not very poor or uneducated so he is equally to blame, making the fault three times.

Incidentally, one of the author's own patients, an educated gentleman from Kerala, employed in a Japanese Company in New Delhi, undergoing maintenance haemodialysis in Batra Hospital, returned to Kerala, his native State, and underwent a paid donor transplant on 23 September 2016 in a hospital at Kochi.[1]

---

[1] References: *TNN* – 4.3.18, *The Hindu* – 3.3.18, *The Indian Express* – 4.3.18, *Deccan Chronicle* – 25.10.17, *The Hindu* – 5.4.14.

HORRIFYING KIDNEY RACKET IN PUNJAB

AMRITSAR

THE SALE AND TRADE OF unrelated kidney transplants have been taking place surreptitiously in Punjab. ever since the 1970s.

It is estimated that nearly 65–70 per cent of the donors in Amritsar are from outside Punjab. Most donors are unrelated to the recipient and are mainly migrant labourers. In some cases, the donors are known to have been kept in captivity until their kidneys were removed.

Surprisingly, the State authorisation committee, headed by the principal of the Government Medical College in Amritsar, had been clearing cases of kidney transplantation in a hackneyed manner, with scant attention to the THOA guidelines. As investigations showed, all donors, coming from outside the State, presented papers showing that they worked as domestic help in the houses of the recipient. This was accepted without question by the 'authorisation committee'. A sizable number of recipients came from as far as Nepal and from outside Punjab and had bogus local addresses. The donors were not local people, and this did not arouse any suspicion in the authorisation committee.

HORRIFYING KIDNEY RACKET IN PUNJAB

> **Rs 100-cr kidney racket busted in Punjab, 2 docs held**
>
> **HT Correspondents**
> *Amritsar/Chandigarh, Jan 12*
>
> THE special investigation team of the Punjab police on Saturday arrested two doctors for their alleged involvement in a kidney racket in Amritsar, which involves an estimated Rs 100 crore.
> According to the investigation report, nearly 65-70 per cent donors and as many recipients of kidneys in Amritsar were from outside Punjab. Most donors were unrelated to the recipients and mainly migrant labourers.

Media reported that the donors had 'offered' to donate their kidneys for 'altruistic' reasons. The clandestine activity of transplantation in Amritsar and Jalandhar had resulted in 20 odd deaths of unidentified donors in the years before 2003. It was a matter of great shame for the medical fraternity in the country and a few doctors and the chairman of the authorisation committee of Amritsar were apprehended in 2003. The middleman was identified and was arrested with two associates and eight 'salesmen' employed to recruit both recipients and donors for this trade in human organs.

It was also alleged that a few donors had actually died due to lack of post-operative care and their bodies were disposed of secretly. Eventually, the vigilance bureau (VB) of Punjab took over the investigations in this kidney racket and of all the related agencies.

The kidney transplant surgeon in the city was arrested, and the Additional Director General of Police and Chief of Special Investigative Team (SIT) called it the 'mother of all scandals in trafficking in human organs'.

For centuries, the holy city of Amritsar had been a centre of reverence, commerce and trade in north India, and this 'unholy' practice of trading human organs and ruthless exploitation of human lives was carried out for years in this holy city by money-hungry professionals and their accomplices.

THE JALANDHAR KIDNEY SCAM

The Transplant Coordinator at the National Kidney Hospital was the key accused in the illegal kidney transplant scam in Jalandhar in 2015.

It is alleged that she was forging documents of illegal donors for money, and a laboratory technician in a private laboratory was accused of changing blood sample reports at the behest of a middleman. Others arrested were from Surya Vihar in New Delhi, two associates from Lucknow and another laboratory technician in Jalandhar. The transplant coordinator of that hospital surrendered on 11 August 2015 and was sent to jail.

The court granted an interim bail to the doctor owner of the National Kidney Hospital and his wife. *'The couple pleaded in the court that as the Jalandhar police officials have absolutely no jurisdiction and power to either investigate or arrest any person for alleged commission of offences under THOA 1994, therefore, the entire proceedings are completely non-est.'* A Special Investigating Team (SIT), headed by ADCP-1 was then assigned to prove the case.

HORRIFYING
KIDNEY
RACKET IN
PUNJAB

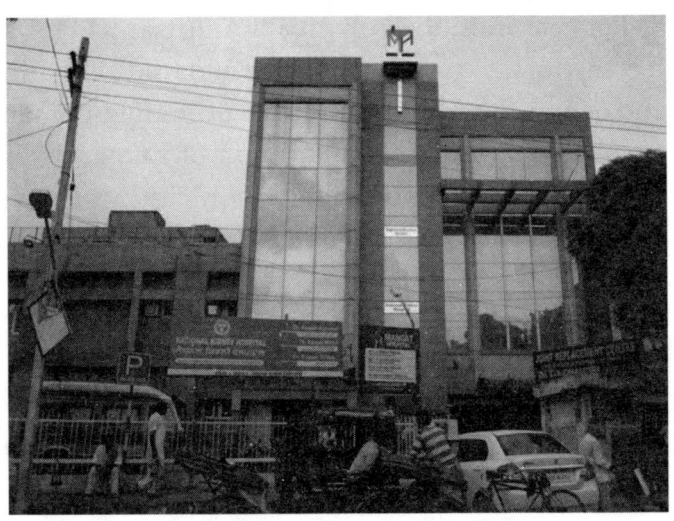

Media image of the National Kidney Hospital involved in the scam.
Source: *Hindustan Times*, 26 March 2016.

Typically, the second-line professionals (the transplant coordinator, laboratory technicians and others who play a big part in any transplant process) were apprehended and put behind bars. However, those who carried out the transplant procedures against the law of the country managed to prove their innocence and escaped legal implications for many years. There were nearly two dozen charge sheets in this case in 2016, and the city police of Jalandhar had submitted a large volume of papers consisting of 855 pages to the court on 25 March 2016.

It is to be noted that the first, original, police SIT did not function for six months and nothing concrete took place in this kidney scam. The government then had to constitute a second SIT to investigate and frame charges against the racketeers.

In the whole picture of rampant kidney transplantation in other cities of Punjab and Haryana, Surya Kidney Centre and Shivalik Hospital in Mohali, it has been alleged that a large number of illegal kidney transplants have been performed in these unknown number of hospitals.

This clandestine practice of kidney transplantation in Punjab was unearthed by the Lucknow police, who investigated the documents in some of their own cases and the role of two hospitals in Mohali on the basis of misleading information by a middleman involved in the Amritsar kidney scam. These hospitals were later given clean chits. So, the discovery of this flourishing racket in kidneys was by accident.[1] The hospitals continue to function.

---

[1] References: *Hindustan Times* – 3.11.13, Webindia 123.com – 12.1.16, *Hindustan Times* – 10.9.15, *The Tribune* – 8.8.15, *The Tribune* – 6.8.15, *Hindustan Times* – 5.10.16, *India News* – 29.12.11.

WEST COAST TO THE EAST

THE GUJARAT KIDNEY SCAM

THE SEEDS OF THE ILLEGAL kidney trade in Gujarat were sown by the infamous Amit Kumar, our Dr K, who had his nefarious activities spread all over the country. His long tentacles reached the impoverished village of Pandoli, where many people's kidneys were taken without their knowledge and against the law of the transplantation act.

The villagers from Pandoli and from some other villages too in the neighbourhood were subjected to ruthless kidney removal at far flung centres such as Dehradun, Uttrakhand, Mumbai, Chennai and Sri Lanka. The middlemen were fellow villagers of Pandoli and other villages, and the kidney racket was extremely well-knit and nearly impregnable. There is no correct estimate as to how many individuals lost their kidneys and in these transactions of millions of rupees, the poor donors received just a few thousand rupees. The 'shark' beneficiaries were the doctors, hospitals and middlemen.

These poor people were taken to Gurgaon, Chennai, and other major cities to undergo the surgical removal of their kidney for transplantation in very rich and connected people across the country and abroad. A victim from this village, 27-year-old Aamir Malek, filed a complaint against the kingpin, middleman and a co-villager for defaulting on a promised big sum of money and not revealing to him that one of his kidneys would be removed.

The Anand police were able to arrest K in Delhi on 29 July 2016 from a Delhi courthouse (Tees Hazari). They also arrested a man identified as 'MCC', alias Mukul, a Valsad-based Ayurveda practitioner; 'SAK' alias Sheru Rehmat Khan Pathan; and a man identified as 'RAV'. The same notorious K had then escaped from police escort in 2016 while travelling on the Swarna Jayanti Express from Delhi to Anand.

It is estimated that more than a dozen men from Pandoli village were duped by middlemen who were residents of the same village. Because the entire scam was done in the Pandoli village, the 'ANAND KIDNEY SCAM' became known as the 'PANDOLI KIDNEY SCAM'.

Some victims, including extremely poor daily wage labourers, were also taken to hospitals in Gujarat. The names of these poor labourers as per police records are Amir Miyan Bannu Miyan Malik, Punambhai Mangalbhai Solanki, Rafiqbhai Ahmad Bhai Vohra, Harshad Bhai Kanubhai Solanki, Ashok Bhai Ambalal Rathor, Narender Punjabhai Solanki, Arvind Ravji Bhai Gohil, Anilbhai Meghajibhai Jhala, Ashokbhai Gordhan Gohil.

Investigative teams were not able to make a headway in other villages as an environment of fear had gripped the entire central part of Gujarat. The trafficked people underwent forensic examination in Ahmedabad Civil Hospital, and it was confirmed that their kidneys were missing.

The reach of the Gujarat scam unravelled when a resident medical officer at the Kidney Hospital in Shahibaug became suspicious of a prospective donor named Mahesh Sharma, who was escorted by a man known as 'SKP', also called Prajapati, who himself had sold his kidney in Nadiad in the past and had made his wife Sajeda undergo removal of her kidney on payment.

On interrogation, SKP admitted that he had been working with a man called 'MJ or Jain' (name changed), a resident of Ratlam in Madhya Pradesh and the two had been working together for the past 11 years, luring organ donors. MJ himself had sold his kidney in Nadiad and had become a racketeer, SKP said.

The modus operandi was to develop a fake relationship with the donor and then get fictitious voter identity cards, birth certificates and other documents of residence etc. of the donor and himself, which were made in Ratlam. SKP lured people who were in urgent need of money and willing to sell their kidneys.

According to police, the accused, Sharma, met his friend 'KP', a resident of Bapunagar, and told him that he urgently needed money. SKP or KP or Prajapati suggested that Sharma sell his kidney and introduced him to a man called Pathan on 8 April 2011. The same day a man called Jain, Pathan and Sharma met at a bhajiya stall near the Civil Hospital in Anand where Jain told Sharma that the total deal would be for ₹2 lakh, of which he would be taking a commission of ₹50,000 for preparing fake documents and setting up the transplant, and ₹10,000 will be paid to Pathan.

Media reports say, on 9 April 2011, all three met once again on the second floor of Bhairunath Parotha House near the Civil Hospital, where they met Dharamchand Bhuralal Jain (51), the patient on dialysis who would be the prospective recipient.

Shortly after, Dharamchand and 'MJ' went to a notary in the Meghaninagar Campus. MJ was introduced as Gyanchand Bhuralal Jain before the notary and necessary documents were produced to show that they were related. The affidavit mentioned that he was the younger brother and was willing to donate his kidney.

A criminal case was filed with the local police and went to the local court. *But in a bizarre development, Amit Kumar's or K's brother, also known as Jeewan Raut (alias Jeevan Kumar, or J Rao), challenged the legality of the probe conducted by Anand police.* So far Amit Kumar or our K had been unconnected with this case.

Ironically, the Gujarat High Court accepted the arguments of his advocate CP (name changed) – that the Centre and the State governments are mandated to appoint an authority under THOA to probe the cases registered under this law. *Section 13 of THOA clearly says that the charges leveled under this Act are to be probed by 'appropriate authority' and the police were/are not the appropriate authority.* The advocate further argued that the Supreme Court, in 2009, had made it clear that police officials are not entitled to probe the offences registered under THOA. Raut approached the court seeking quashing of the investigation after police authorities allegedly started building pressure on him during the probe.[1]

IN ODISHA, WELFARE SECRETARY OR KIDNEY TOUT?

In May 2014, in a nursing home called Sukanya, in Badambadi, Odisha illegal kidney transplants were conducted, and donors were lured there from Kendrapara. It took three years for the police to gather all the information and file charges.

A 39-year-old man, Ramesh Chand Sahu, a guard in a private company at Kalinganagar, alleged that he was lured to sell his kidney in a corporate hospital at Vasant Kunj in Delhi. He was escorted by several touts who he identified as 'T Khan', 'F Tandi' and 'N Sahu' in March 2011. Upon reaching Delhi, Ramesh Sahu complained of abdominal pain after a drink and was admitted in the said hospital. He was told that he had a kidney stone while in the hospital and that his kidney matched with some rich individual's.

Sahu was subsequently persuaded to donate a kidney in exchange of a large sum of money. After the

---

[1] References: *Ahmedabad Mirror* – 22.5.11.

operation, he was given ₹1 lakh and promised more, and he was kept in a rented accommodation for a few days before being sent to Bhubaneswar. Upon asking for the rest of the promised money of ₹5 lakh, he was threatened with dire consequences and harm to his mother living alone in their native village.

In May 2014, three people, including a woman named Sharmistha, were arrested on a complaint by Padmini Nayak, a resident of Nayak Sahi in the slums in Mangalabag, Cuttack. She complained that 'dalals' had created a false income certificate to facilitate a kidney donation in her case. 'While our family income is no more than ₹100 per day, I was told to say that my income is ₹2.5 lakh in a month.' Not only was the income certificate false, even Padmini's photograph was morphed with the family members of the kidney recipient to prove that she is related to the family.

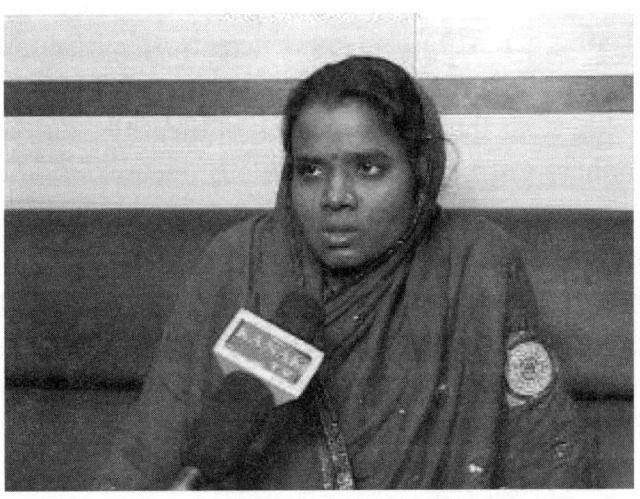

Padmini Nayak talking to Kanak TV.

Padmini was trapped by 'madam' Sharmistha (Nayak) who was working as secretary of a Mahila Samiti, a Self Help Group (SHG) in Mangalabag area of Cuttack. Sharmistha had been visiting Padmini's house frequently and talking about her financial troubles and ultimately proposed to Padmini that she sell one of her kidneys for ₹3 lakh. Padmini was assured of care after the surgery at Apollo Hospital, Bhubaneshwar. At the time of discharge from the hospital, she was paid by Sharmistha ₹2 lakh instead of ₹3 lakh as assured in the deal. This made Padmini realise that she had been duped and she complained to the police.

It is also shameful that the secretary of a Self Help Group (SHG) became an active contributor in the illegal trade and brought infamy to the SHG movement in the State.[2]

TELANGANA: DROUGHT-HIT DONORS

In 2002, at the Government General Hospital, Guntur the authorisation committee suspected a kidney racket from the impersonation of identities on the Aadhaar Card and other fictitious documents of a prospective kidney donor from Durgi Mandal in the impoverished region of Palnadu.

It may be recalled that there were reports of a large number of cases involving distress sale of kidneys in the drought-hit Palnadu area in the year 2002. Clearly, a gang was involved.

[2] References: *The Odisha Bulletin* – 26.5.14, *The Times of India* – 7.6.14, *Odisha Sun Times* Bureau – 13.5.14.

Two other cases were unravelled at Narsaraopet. In this case, it appeared that a Mandal revenue officer and some middlemen were also caught, and ironically, the tehsildar had himself lodged a complaint with the Narsaraopet town police.

A man named Naik, who was arrested in 2015 on the charge of fabricating his Aadhaar card, revealed the modus operandi of the gang operating in 2015. The four accused were kingpin 'KBR', two men identified as 'INR' and 'AY', and another man named NP Babu alias Bobby (all names appear to be fictitious) from Tenali.

Man Allegedly Tries To Sell Kidney With Fake Aadhaar In Andhra Pradesh

| Updated: January 04, 2018 16:09 IST

In February 2015, in yet another incident, the Telangana police had busted a racket involving a multi-crore international kidney transplant trade. Two men, identified as DC and SP (names changed), were arrested for having admitted to giving medical checkups to test for preliminary kidney compatibility to over a hundred people from Delhi, Andhra Pradesh and Tamil Nadu at a diagnostic laboratory. The selected donors were sent to Sri Lanka after a primary health checkup at Ahmedabad, which had become the hub for illegal transplant operations, the arrested men told the police.

The surgeries were done at Nawalok Hospital, Western Hospital and Lankan Hospital in Colombo, they said.

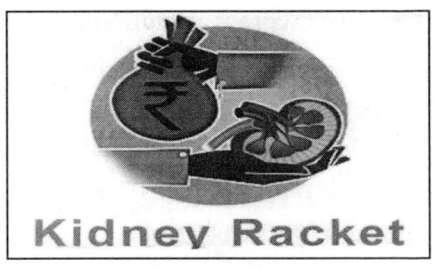

WEST COAST TO THE EAST

Suraj (name changed), a hotel management student, was introduced to an agent on a website facilitating kidney donation, and after selling his kidney in 2014 for ₹5 lakh, he became the principal agent who arranged passports and visas for illegal donors sent to hospitals in Colombo.

The impoverished donors were from different parts of the country; four were from Nalgonda district, four from Hyderabad, four from Bangalore, two from Tamil Nadu and one each from Delhi and Mumbai. The medical investigations of these donors were done in Mumbai and Ahmedabad. Suraj was arrested with a man called AH alias Qasim, and two others named as Mahesh and Naresh from Nalgonda.

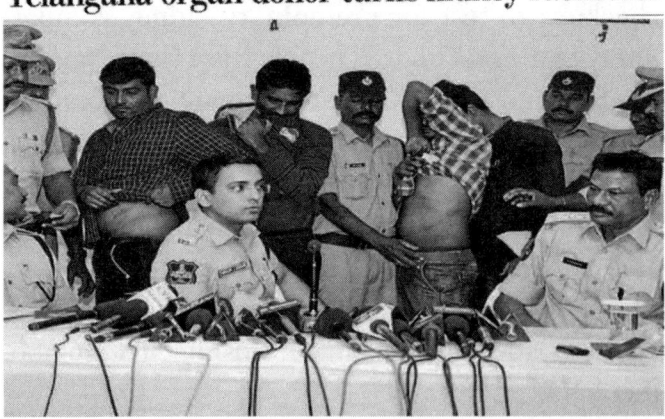

HYDERABAD – WHISTLEBLOWER DOCTOR

A former Medical Director of a private hospital called Continental Hospital in Gachibowli, in the border district of Andhra Pradesh, had himself lodged a complaint in 2016 that during his tenure in the hospital, there were 'certain acts of wrongdoing' in kidney transplant cases.

He said, initially, the Hospital Internal Transplant Committee had rejected a case where they thought the donor and the recipient were 'not biologically related'. But the same panel had approved two other cases by forging the signatures of the Medical Director who then took up the role of a whistle blower in November 2016.

STATE CADAVER ORGAN TRANSPLANTATION AUTHORITY (JEEVAN DAAN)

Jeevan Daan, the State Cadaver Organ Transplantation Authority, was set up in undivided Andhra Pradesh in 2013. Since then, the organisation has been able to obtain organs from 241 brain-dead patients and nearly 1,000 patients have been beneficiaries.

Ironically, they were unable to convince a single Muslim about the need for organ donation and were unable to integrate hospitals run by minorities to be part of their network. Religious beliefs and objection to organ donation was cited.[3]

---

[3] References:
   The Hindu – Guntur, January 26, 2018 – http://www.thehindu.com
   The New Indian Express, 26th January 2018 – http://www.newindianexpress.com
   India: https://www.hindustantimes.com/india

IN THE HEARTLAND OF MP, BIHAR, UP

FREE MEDICAL CHECK UP – KIDNEY LOST

THE CITY OF UJJAIN HAS a very high religious significance and is considered one of the prime places of the Shani deity, besides its Kal Bhairav temple to Mahadeva, one of the trinities of the Hindu pantheon. A large number of Hindus in the country and abroad go to this temple town to worship and ward off the negative effects of Lord Shani.

In June 2008, an illegal kidney racket was busted in this town where four suspects were arrested during the search operations conducted by police on the eve of the visit of the President of India, Pratibha Patil.

A man named 'S' from Nadiad, and 'V Patel' of Ahmedabad were considered the masterminds behind the racket and had local contacts in Ujjain. They motivate poor people in government hospitals to move to hospitals allied to Starlink Hospital in Ahmedabad and to hospitals in Chennai, Coimbatore and Indore on the pretext of getting them 'better treatment' free of cost.

The arrested men had admitted to the police that at least 15 kidneys had been removed illegally at these centres. The *'Better Treatment Without Payment'* had included the removal of a kidney. These poor people were sent home with paltry amounts for their kidneys.[1]

Kidney racket busted in Madhya Pradesh

An illegal kidney trade racket has been busted in Madhya Pradesh's Ujjain town, say the police.

INDIA (HTTPS://WWW.HINDUSTANTIMES.COM/INDIA/) Updated: Jun 28, 2008 15:14 IST

BIHAR – ILLEGAL KIDNEY REMOVAL

Though there has been no report of organised illegal trade of kidneys leading to scams in the State of Bihar, there have been media reports of donors from Bihar being taken to Punjab, Gurgaon and other transplant centres in the country for kidney donation for money.

Yet another kidney racket in Bihar, NBW issued against medic

In December 2005, it was reported in the local media that 30-year-old Surender, a rickshaw-puller, had *both his kidneys removed* at an unregistered private clinic at Mahnar, Vaishali district of Bihar and was shifted to the Patna Medical College and Hospital (PMCH) where he died. It is unknown if his kidneys were removed for illegal kidney transplantation.[2]

---

[1] Reference: *Hindustan Times* – Saturday, August 11, 2018.
[2] References: *India News – The Times of India* – 23.12.05, zeenews.india.com – 23.12.05, *The Hindu* – 25.12.05.

UTTAR PRADESH KIDNEY SCAM

In 2004, two touts, identified as PR and VK (name changed), were arrested by the Delhi Police in connection with the illegal kidney removals at the Noida Medical Centre. However, both were later released.

Media reports said at the time that 12 such cases had taken place in the Noida Medical Centre, 3 in a central Delhi hospital and 2 in another prominent hospital in South Delhi. The metropolitan magistrate in Delhi had at that time issued notices to prominent hospitals in the city under a cloud of suspicion.

Until then, there had been no reports of big kidney scandals or scams in the largest State of India, Uttar Pradesh. On account of meager facilities of transplantation available to vast number of kidney failure patients, there had been very few sporadic news items in the media in this matter.

The great 'mafia boss' of kidney agents – the same 'PR' who owns a 'tree-house' in the outskirts in Kolkata – charged and arrested for the kidney scam in Apollo Hospital in Delhi in May 2016, had surfaced in Kanpur in 2018.

If true, the scandal came to the notice of the police after a woman called Sunita – wife of an electrician called Rajesh Kumar Kashyap in Kanpur – was lured by this gang of six touts, with the promise of a job in Delhi. In a well-planned operation, one of the touts got the couple Rajesh and Sunita into a hotel in Delhi and Sunita underwent blood tests in a Delhi hospital. She was told that her prospective employer is a well-to-do person and that she would have to cook meals and would be employed only after a medical checkup, which is the norm in Delhi's job market.

Later, this Sunita was assured a sum of ₹40 lakh, media reports said. Out of this, she was given ₹3 lakh as advance money. In addition, her name was changed to a Muslim name and her Aadhaar Card was quickly changed in an outlet in Delhi. Suspecting fraud, Sunita and her husband returned to Kanpur and filed a police complaint. This is how this kidney scandal unfolded and six touts were arrested.

On intense interrogation by the police, the middlemen admitted that they have facilitated twelve transplants in this manner so far.

Delhi doctor handled international buyers

Media reports in 2019 said, this gang had been operating from Kanpur, Lucknow, Agra, Meerut, Noida and New Delhi.

In this interstate kidney scandal, a Delhi-based private practitioner is said to be handling the gang's international clientele. Police say that this multi-crore illegal trade has been flourishing for over five years.

According to the Kanpur SSP, doctors have been playing a key role in arranging tourist visas of donors who were then sent to Sri Lanka and Turkey for transplantation.

At this stage a gang of six agents is in police custody. These members are found to have links to technicians and paramedics in specific hospitals, report the national newspapers. *The Times of India*[3] of 20 February 2019 says:

---

[3] References: *Amar Ujala* – 18.2.19 *Navbharat Times* – 18.2.19 *Jagran* – 18.2.19 *The Times of India* – 20.2.19 *The Times of India* – 28.2.19.

The kingpin would hold classes of prospective donors at a rented accommodation in Delhi to remove concerns about post-surgery complications. To stamp out suspicion, he would coach the donors to say they were voluntarily donating kidneys out of affection to the recipient.

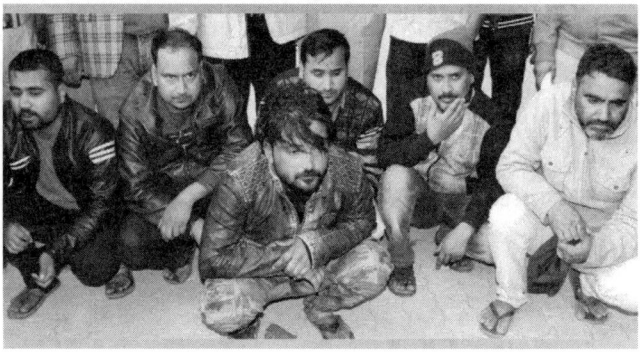

IN THE HEARTLAND OF MP, BIHAR, UP

KIDNEY SCAMS IN DELHI

IN THE CAPITAL OF THE country, with premiere medical institutes such as AIIMS and Safdarjung Hospital, as well as it being the seat of the union government with conglomerate of VIPs, constantly there is a heterogeneous composition of patients.

There is also always a heavy influx of patients coming from northern provinces and neighbouring countries of Nepal, Afghanistan and Bangladesh. The facilities of dialysis and transplant, however, were in the early years available only at AIIMS, Delhi and PGI, Chandigarh.

The annual grant for kidney services, including dialysis and transplantation, was a meager ₹90,000 at AIIMS in the 1970s and '80s.

In the early seventies, the immunosuppressive drugs for transplantation had included Prednisolone, Azathioprine and Cyclosporine. Cadaveric transplantation, or transplantation from dead bodies, was non-existent across the nation except in one or two cases from Mumbai, which were unsuccessful.

In the beginning, the majority of transplants were done from an immediate related family source. The unrelated cases were also from the extended family circle. Despite good and compatible donor selection, there were still 'disguised donors' from outer family groups. The second kidney transplant at AIIMS was a 'paid unrelated donor' under the care of this author who never returned for follow-up at all. This was before the country had any organ donation law.

Those days, there was no need for any documentary evidence of relationships, and all statements made by recipient and donor were accepted by the medical teams. There were umpteen complications in both the recipient and the donor, yet the transplant activities gained momentum at both centres. There were no so-called 'scams', no middleman and there was an atmosphere of tranquility and satisfaction at these centres, in Delhi, Chandigarh, Mumbai and at CMC Vellore. The total number of transplants had remained small and there were plenty of prospective recipients. The dialysis facilities for long-term treatment were not available, and it was a common occurrence that patients were refused dialysis.

Many left to die for want of dialysis

Hindustan Times, 24 August 1982.

In this scene of insufficient equipment, untrained manpower and poor facilities, there was an accelerated development of dialysis centres in other major hospitals in the country. But transplantation was still only possible at hospitals in Delhi, Chandigarh, Mumbai and Vellore, and the number of transplants remained miniscule.

Subsequently, there was a gradual increase of activity in renal transplants in multiple centres in Mumbai, Chennai, Kolkata and Hyderabad. In these centres, the transplants were performed from related donors and the total number started increasing in early eighties.

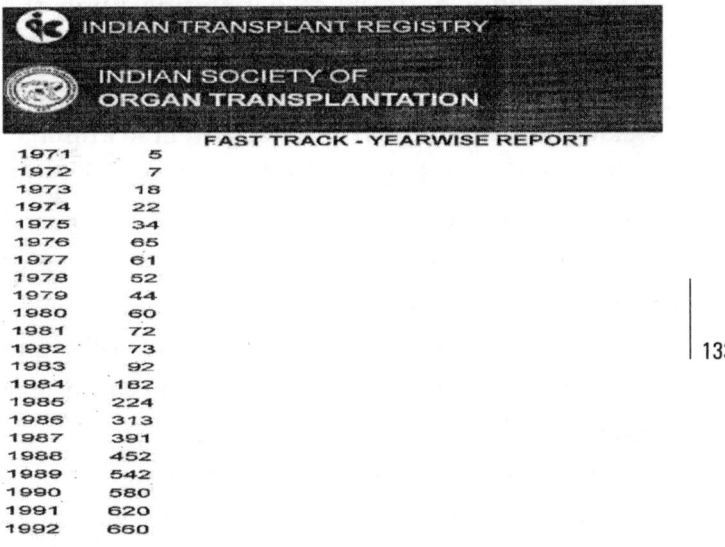

Year	Number
1971	5
1972	7
1973	18
1974	22
1975	34
1976	65
1977	61
1978	52
1979	44
1980	60
1981	72
1982	73
1983	92
1984	182
1985	224
1986	313
1987	391
1988	452
1989	542
1990	580
1991	620
1992	660

Total number of Transplants from 1971 to 1992 – 4,569.

Rich patients and those whose expenditures were paid for by the government went abroad for transplants, but their numbers were very small.

The number of unrelated kidney donors increased even when related donors were possible, as the families of recipients were pressured to choose and favour unrelated sources for transplantation. As the word spread of successful kidney transplantation even with 'unrelated' donors, medical teams and transplant surgeons themselves advised recipients for unrelated kidney donors.

The 'ethical versus unethical' practice of transplantation was debated among medical professionals, and it was considered that unrelated transplantation was not desirable, despite the medical professional's advise. By then, the trade of kidneys was well established, and a kidney from an unrelated source commanded a hefty price depending upon the economic status and anxiety of a recipient's family.

Patients from Delhi and other northern regions seeking unrelated donors invariably went to Mumbai, as it was easy to locate a middleman and willing doctors for transplants. Some patients chose Chennai and Vellore, depending upon the convenience of family and relative's advice.

In Delhi, 'free-wheeling' agents were not visible and were relatively behind-the-scenes. Organisations like Lok Kalyan Samiti were allegedly working to procure unrelated and poor kidney donors. There were anonymous individuals who played the role of middlemen, and their identities were never divulged as they were accepted as cousins in Delhi and Chandigarh.

> The going rate in cases of organised sale varies from forty thousand to seventy thousand, depending on the urgency and desperation of the recipient.

Sunday Magazine, 22 December 1985.

My colleague, Dr RVS Yadav, a pioneering surgeon in the country, was invited from Chandigarh by Batra Hospital in Delhi to start a kidney transplant programme there in 1989.

Over a period of four years, this hospital became the only centre in Delhi other than AIIMS, performing kidney transplantation. By the beginning of 1990, Dr Yadav and I, as the only nephrologists in the country's capital city and both aware of the flourishing kidney bazaars in the country, were mulling legislation on organ donation, convinced that cadaver transplant could easily replace live kidney transplants in the country; we were a country teeming with people and our daily deaths too were many. We had first suggested laws on organ donations in the 1970s but now we felt the urgent need to push for it.

However, by 1992, I realised that there was a sudden change in the transplant activity in Delhi. I then discovered that a small hospital called Parmarth Mission Hospital had started doing kidney transplantations as well.

This was an unregistered nursing home, which illegally took electricity from overhead transmission lines. This nursing home used 'unrelated' donors. All laboratory work, including HLA typing, was carried out at a central laboratory in Connaught Place, the central shopping centre in Delhi. A nephrologist was also working at Parmarth Mission Hospital at that time.

An educated man, named Virender Gupta, was apprehended by the police, when this racket was exposed. He was responsible for the 'unrelated paid' transplantation at that hospital. Media reports at that time said, Gupta was the kingpin for unrelated paid donors – he was the supply chain manager for donors and had supplied 125 donors to hospitals all over the country.

Gupta had a BA degree from Madhya Pradesh and was unable to find a suitable job in Punjab. He then went to Mumbai, where he unsuccessfully tried to sell one of his own kidneys. After his 'unsuccess' in Mumbai, he traveled to Delhi and started a kidney trade with a few of his trusted friends.

Gupta operated from a chemist shop in Jahangirpuri locality in Delhi and resided in Adarsh Nagar. He had sent donors to Mumbai and lesser-known hospitals and nursing homes in Chennai, Amritsar and even Noida in Uttar Pradesh. The donors were scouted from various blood banks in New Delhi, the Walled City and Connaught Place. The price of a donor was ₹30,000 to ₹70,000. To paid donors, blood banks offered ₹30 for one session of blood donation, as in Kolkata and elsewhere in the country. In those days, voluntary blood donation camps by the general public were not popular, unlike now. Nor did hospitals have donor registries. The regular donors to the blood banks were very poor and destitute, mostly men who needed ready cash for alcohol and daily sustenance.

The kidney trade flourished smoothly until a donor, a drug addict, Pradeep Kumar was lured into selling his kidney for ₹30,000. While he was at a de-addiction centre, Santulan, in West Delhi, his father was told by the de-addiction centre to lodge a complaint with the police that Pradeep had been drugged and forced to sign an affidavit agreeing to donate his kidney and a transplant was done from him in May 1992 at the Parmarth Mission Hospital.

The agent or middleman named was Virender Gupta who had lured Pradeep into drugs. At that time, the police turned away the father, a mill worker, on the grounds that 'no offence' had been committed under the Indian Penal Code by the agent. Someone went to the media.

The national newspaper *The Indian Express* splashed a big news item – of a flourishing kidney trade in July 1992 and highlighted the kidney transplant of a drug addict.

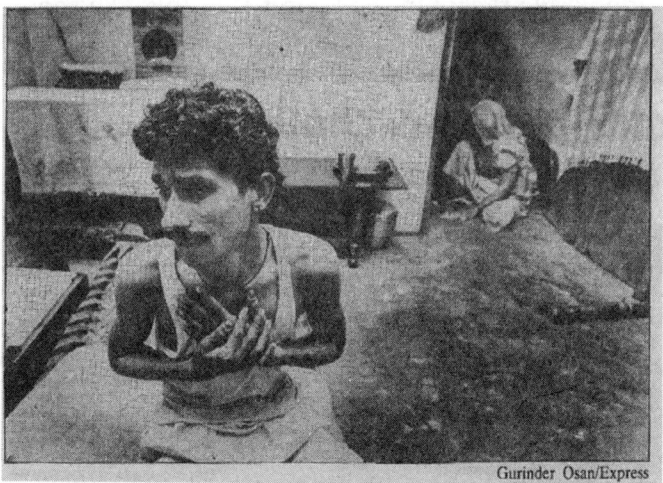

Gurinder Osan/Express

Commercial transactions by living donors of their organs hit the headlines when racketeers made Pradip Kumar part with his kidney for some 'smack'. But is selling one's non-renewable tissue illegal ? More importantly, if it is legal now, would it become illegal once the Bill becomes an Act ? This is just one of the many aspects that the Bill is ambiguous about.

At this point, the President of the Delhi High Court Bar Association took up the case and public sentiments were aroused against this commercial harvesting of kidneys from unrelated donors. The matter was also raised in Parliament by a few members in July 1992. The time was ripe at last for forcing through some laws.

On 17 September 1992, the Delhi High Court issued notices to the Union Ministers of Home, Health and Family Welfare and the Lt-Governor and Police Commissioner of Delhi. A petition filed sought prosecution of the concerned doctors and officials of Parmarth Mission Hospital, along with the broker of the kidney scandal.

Following Delhi High Court's intervention, a committee headed by the Secretary of Delhi administration began an in-depth probe and scrutiny of the kidney sale racket in the Union Territory. The committee visited two private hospitals and extensively scrutinised the hospital records, interviewed doctors and hospital managers and finally concluded that the news items had a 'very sound basis'.

The committee also recommended that the government urgently create ways and means to put a stop to such operations where human organs were supplied as commodities for pecuniary gains. The members of this committee also gave a clean chit to Batra Hospital, one of the few private facilities offering kidney transplants in the city at that time.

However, this was not the end of the saga of kidney sales in Delhi. On 5 March 1993, the *Indian Express* newspaper again published a front-page news story headlined 'Kidney Racket Kingpin Nabbed'. There were certain arrests and anticipatory bails granted.

In a night-long operation, Virender Gupta had been arrested after police spoke to his 'friends' over the phone, posing as a potential kidney customer. His accomplices including the doctors involved and some agents were promptly nabbed.

The writ petition in the Delhi High Court was filed by the Delhi Nashabandi Samiti, the de-addition organisation. They had also written open letters to various dignitaries and began a campaign against unrelated kidney harvest.

The print media also worked overtime. Statements and opinions of legal, moral and ethical consideration and justification were expressed. Hindi language newspapers, periodicals and the national newspaper, *The Hindu*, had all highlighted the details of this scandal.

With this ongoing huge media coverage, *surprisingly the medical fraternity, Delhi Medical Association and the Delhi branch of Indian Medical Association, took a very strong stand on behalf of the kidney surgeons and nephrologists involved, and they demanded immediate release of the detained doctors.*

Bail for surgeon in kidney sale case

चिकित्सकों ने गुर्दा प्रत्यारोपण बंद करने की धमकी दी

डांक्टर की गिरफ्तारी के विरोध में डायलिसिस रोकी

The Parmarth Mission Hospital, however, was eventually indicted by the court for running a hospital without permission and carrying on purchased unrelated kidney transplants.

At this stage, I began to consistently appeal for a legislation on organ donation and transplant. I and my colleagues vociferously argued from every platform available to us that there was an urgent need to enact legislation to monitor organ transplants and do away with commercial exploitation of the poor, the malnourished and addicted-to-drugs donors. We believed that laws could and would stop the 'rampant live unrelated' donor exploitation and stop sale and purchase of live kidneys.

> **KIDNEY SCAMS IN DELHI**
>
> Dr Ramesh Kumar, head of the nephrology department of Batra Hospital, New Delhi, is convinced of the need to watch over organ transplants and do away with commercial exploitation. Many of those who sell kidney, he says, are unhealthy or addicted to drugs. He, however, finds no harm in transplants as such since "there is nothing life-threatening in donating a kidney". He has, incidentally, protested the Doordarshan telecast of *Saheb*, the Anil Kapoor-Amrita Singh tearjerker about an upcoming footballer who sells his kidney to marry off his sister, sacrificing his sports career. "The brother of one of my patients, who was willing to donate a kidney, backed out after seeing that film!" he says angrily.
>
> THE WEEK ■ NOV. 8, 1992

Those were early days for colour television in India too. A strong protest was voiced against the telecast of the Bollywood film, *Saheb*, telecast by the government channel Doordarshan. The film depicted an up-and-coming football player who sacrifices his sports career by selling one of his kidneys to marry off his sister. This film portrays kidney transplantation in a negative light, and after watching this film, the brother of one of my patients backed out of donating one of his kidneys to his sister. There is nothing wrong in kidney transplant, as such. Nor in any other organ transplant. It is the commercialisation that is wrong.

A comprehensive human organ transplant Act was urgently required and the author mobilised the medical community in Delhi to request the Union government to take positive steps at an early date.[1] Today, India has a very specific law. But our expectations have been belied.

A law needs very strict implementation.

When there is social sanction to buying 'unrelated' kidney and not to cadaver organs or donations from relatives, no amount of laws can control the bazaars for organs operating in India. The Indian rupee in August 2019 was the lowest currency in Asia. When just a few thousands of this rupee matters so much even today that a man or woman is ready to sell his kidney, we can no longer say 'an uneducated poor has been duped' and shrug of social responsibility. Awareness and ethics are both lacking, and that trade in live kidneys continues in India two decades into the 21st century says much about us Indians.

THE APOLLO SCAM

It was a chance happening that attracted the attention of the police on duty outside Apollo Hospital,

---

[1] References: *Hindustan Times* – 24.8.1982; *Sunday Magazine* – 22.12.1985; *The Indian Express* – July, 1992; *The Week* – 8.11.1992.

Delhi on 2nd June 2016. A woman by the name Mamta (name changed), wife of a tout named Devender (name changed), was in a heated exchange with her husband in the foyer of the hospital for cheating her out of the amount received after one of her kidneys was sold.

On interrogation, the woman revealed that her husband, a native of New Jalpaiguri, West Bengal, had forced Mamta to donate her kidney a month before this racket came to light. They were taken to the police station at Sarita Vihar, New Delhi, where Mamta told the police that her husband had promised her ₹3 lakh for one of her kidneys. She had agreed to do so, but she had received only ₹1.5 lakh from the middleman and she had been angry.

KIDNEY SCAMS IN DELHI

Domestic strife gave police a whiff of racket

Kidney racket busted in Delhi; prominent multispeciality hospital under lens

On the basis of this information from this woman, two senior doctors of Apollo Hospital were questioned in connection to this kidney trading racket, and they were asked to join in the probe under CRPC section 160 of this matter. Three other doctors, who were members of the hospital-based authorisation committee, were also asked to join in the investigations and to verify documents pertaining to the transplant.

All the 13 people involved in the case, including hospital secretaries, middlemen, a kingpin (let us call him PR), a few donors and one recipient, were interrogated in the widespread investigation process undertaken by a special investigation team (SIT) of the Delhi police. This 43-year-old kingpin, PR, was believed to be associated with similar rackets in Nepal, Sri Lanka and Indonesia and was apprehended in West Bengal. He had been under police observation for operating similar rackets in Jalandhar, Coimbatore and Hyderabad.

The modus operandi of this kidney racket was quite standard, where a donor was shown as a 'relative' or 'spouse' of the recipient on the basis of forged documents. The local tout was constantly in touch with the secretarial staff in the nephrology department of Apollo Hospital to arrange a suitable donor on a payment of ₹3 to ₹5 lakh. The recipient was typically charged between ₹25 to ₹30 lakh.

This racket came under police scanner since June 2016 and investigators soon learnt that multiple transplants had been done under its scheme, *after an internal competent authority had approved the presented documentation.* In this widespread saga, the police arrested not only Mamta and her husband, but also another woman identified as a kidney donor associated with the racket. In a spree of arrests, a 22-year-old kidney recipient was also arrested, and his bail was rejected, because he had knowingly participated in the transplantation process, which prima facie appeared to be a 'pre-planned criminal conspiracy'.

Among the arrested were several touts, the kingpin and an associate from Kanpur who himself had donated his kidney in 2014. Another tout, who was the coordinator of the gang responsible for lodging the donors, laboratory tests, interaction with recipient and hospital staff, and negotiations for money, was also arrested. The Joint Commissioner of Police (southeast range) said that at the end of July 2017, the police had arrested 13 people, while four others had surrendered. Among those arrested, two were secretarial staff in the nephrology department of Apollo Hospital.

Police formed a special investigation team with twenty-five members to crack the entire nexus of hospital-recipient-middlemen-donor. A 1,316-page charge sheet by the Delhi police charged 17 people under various sections of the Indian Penal Code and relevant sections of THOA. Besides invoking sections 120-b (conspiracy), 419 (cheating by impersonation), 420 (cheating), 467 (forgery), 468 (forgery for purpose of cheating) and 471 (using forged documents as genuine) of the IPC, Sections 18, 19 and 20 of the THOA that deal with the consequences of violating the act have also been used.

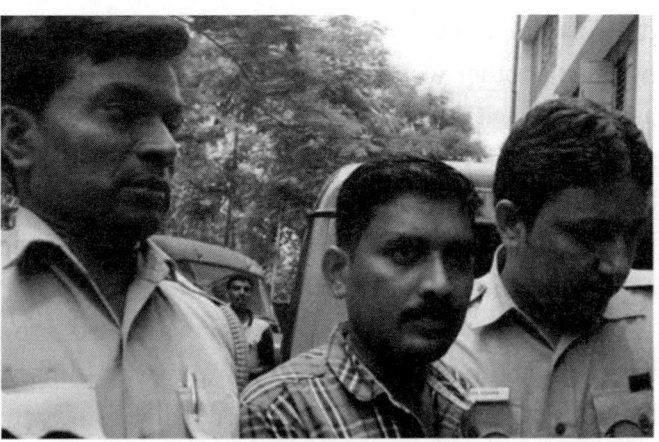

The kingpin involved in the Apollo scam.

The kingpin, the mafia boss PR, had a well-established network of kidney trade in the country, police said. He had confessed to the police that the racket spanned several countries including Sri Lanka, Indonesia and Singapore and involved middlemen, organ donors and their recipients and that he and his team of accomplices had ensured over 100 recipients who had received illegal kidney donations.

PR travelled abroad looking for kidney recipients and had bought a 'tree-house' for himself in Kolkata. One of these houses was bought for over ₹1 crore and was located close to the Kolkata airport. At the time of his arrest, he told the police that 'he was in touch with 25 recipients and had taken advances from them'. It is well known that the 'kidney touts' roam around the labour markets in the poorest districts of Bihar, West Bengal, Uttar Pradesh, Tamil Nadu and Delhi in search of potential donors, the media reported.

Information was received that the members of the gang would come to Apollo Hospital on 2 June 2017 to hold a meeting between a donor and relatives of a recipient. A raid was conducted, and four touts were caught as disclosed by CP (southeast), New Delhi.

A senior nephrologist at the All India Institute of Medical Sciences believed a kidney racket of such a magnitude, cutting across several States, could not take place without the knowledge of managers at a hospital and senior doctors.[2] On the other hand, a senior transplant surgeon at Apollo Hospital stated that 'we are doctors, not an investigating agency. We have to go by the documents that have been

---

[2] https://www.rediff.com/news/report/apollo-kidney-racket-is-the-tip-of-the-iceberg/20160615.htm – June 7, 2016.

placed before us. We do not have the wherewithal to check their veracity'. As such, the very purpose of competent authority of hospital and hospital-based authorisation committee consisting of two senior appointees of the Government of Delhi was defeated in the process of impersonation of donors and submitted fictitious documents, the media reported.

Apollo Kidney Racket: Senior Doctor's Assistant Arrested

Apollo kidney racket: Kingpin arrested; 10 docs to be quizzed

Police busts kidney racket, 2 staffers of top Delhi hospital among 5 arrested

Apollo Hospital's statement on the kidney racket was:

KIDNEY SCAMS IN DELHI

The police approached us yesterday afternoon for their investigation in the matter pertaining to an alleged kidney sale racket. We are cooperating and providing to them all information required to help them in their investigation. This matter is of grave concern and our teams are extending all support to the police.

The hospital, in order to ensure compliance with the law and diligence in process has an independent body with external members also for according consent for any transplant surgery. This committee goes through all documents necessary to ensure that requirements under the act are complied with. Further, the hospital has ensured that all due process as per the law has been followed.

The police in their investigation has identified secretarial staff of some doctors, who are not employees of the hospital, who have been involved in the alleged racket. While all due precautions were conducted, the use of fake and forged documents was used for this racket with a criminal intent. The hospital has been a victim of a well-orchestrated operation to cheat patients and the hospital. We urge the police to take the strictest of action against all those involved. Indraprastha Apollo Hospitals has always abided by the law with utmost care and diligence and shall continue to do so.

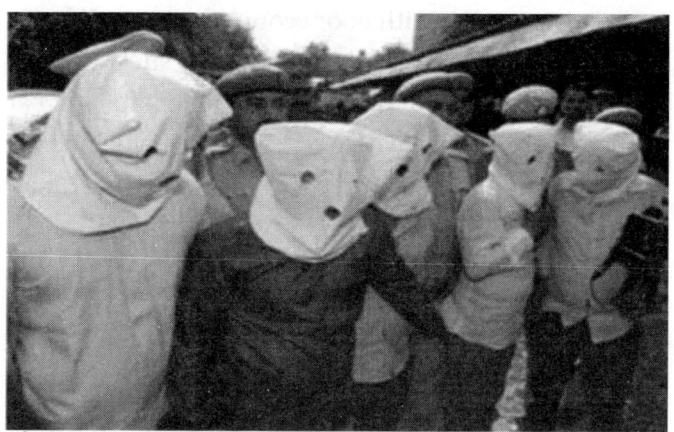

Five people arrested in the Apollo hospital kidney scam in Delhi. This is a media video grab.

In 2017, the special investigation team arrested two other people for allegedly receiving kidneys through an illegal organ donation racket, which was busted in June of the previous year. The Deputy Commissioner of Police (southeast district) said that two other kidney recipients had been identified as Aggarwal and Gupta. 'While one paid ₹3 lakh to Rao (a middleman) and ₹8 lakh for medical expenses, the other paid ₹2 lakh to Rao and ₹8 lakh for medical expenses. Gupta came into contact with Rao through the personal assistant of a senior doctor, while Aggarwal was put in touch with a tout through personal secretaries of doctors at Apollo Hospital.' A former personal secretary from Apollo hospital, New Delhi was also apprehended.

A scam was busted through an undercover operation of the crime branch of the Delhi police at the same time at Batra Hospital, New Delhi, where the modus operandi was similar, and masterminds were different.

The donors were scouted from West Bengal, Eastern UP and other parts of the country – all found from communities with poor economic status. It is not beyond the imagination of anyone that such a racket is impossible without involvement of hospital staff at different levels as the whole process of transplantation is a coordinated teamwork. In 2018, the Hyderabad police busted a kidney racket by arresting a Shirdi-based doctor for selling a 'kidney package' for ₹30 lakh, arranging donors, and taking patients abroad for surgery. In Jalandhar, a 'terror alert' led to the unravelling of a kidney racket in the previous year.

KIDNEY SCAMS IN DELHI

Following the Apollo exposure, the Delhi government passed an order suspending the license of Indraprastha Apollo Hospital to conduct transplant for three months – until 5 January 2018. However, in the interest of patients, the government had allowed operation for cases approved by the hospital-based authorisation committee prior to issuance of the order. This spurred investigations across hospitals in Delhi and around the country. Shares of Apollo Hospitals Enterprises dropped 2% on a winter Friday to close the BSE, where the benchmark Sensex ended 0.5% lower.[3]

[3] References: *Hindustan Times* (http://paper.hindustantimes.com) – August 24, 2018;
http://www.rediff.com/news/report/apollo-kidney-racket – June 15, 2016;
http://timesofindia.indiatimes.com/city/delhi/kidney-racket – June 4, 2016;
http://economictimes.indiatimes.com/news/politics-and-nation – June 7, 2016;

THE BATRA HOSPITAL SCAM: FICTITIOUS IDENTITY AND MAKEOVER

Twenty-third of May 2017 was a dark day in the previously unblemished track record of kidney transplantation in Batra Hospital since 1989.

I had started the services of Nephrology, Haemodialysis, Peritoneal dialysis, Continuous Ambulatory Peritoneal Dialysis (CAPD), Kidney Transplantation at AIIMS in 1973, Sir Ganga

---

http://www.ndtv.com/delhi/news/kidney-racket-delhi – June 28, 2016;

http://www.firstpost.com/india/apollo-hospital-kidney-racket – June 8, 2016;

http://www.straitstimes.com/asia/south-asia/top-indian-hospital – June 5, 2016;

http://www.ndtv.com/delhi-news/apollo-kidney-racket – June 12, 2016;

http://economictimes.indiatimes.com/news/potitics-and-nation – June 11, 2016;

http://timesofindia.indiatimes.com/city/delhi/2-bihar-kidney-donors – May 28, 2017;

http://www.ndtv.com/delhi-news/kidney-racket-busted-in-delhis – June 4, 2016;

http://www.dnaindia.com/india/report-police-charge-sheet-17 – September 2, 2016;

http://www.indiatoday.in/india/story/5-including-2-staff-of-top – June 3, 2016;

http://post.jagran.com/kidney-racket-busted-in-delhi-prominent – June 4, 2016;

http://www.ndtv.com/delhi-news/kidney-racket-2-senior-doctors – July 13, 2016;

http://medicaldialogues.in/apollo-kidney-racket-sit-gets – November 12, 2016;

http://indianexpress.com/article/india/india-news-india/delhi – November 11, 2016;

http://timesofindia.indiatimes.com/city/delhi/kidney-racket – June 4, 2016;

https://www.thehindu.com/news/cities/Delhi/Kidney-trade-racket-busted-at-South-Delhi-Hospital/article14382481.ece; June 3, 2016 updated October 18, 2016.

Ram Hospital in 1984 and at Batra Hospital & Medical Research Centre in 1987. My esteemed colleague Dr RVS Yadav from PGI, Chandigarh had joined Batra Hospital while on sabbatical leave in 1989 for one year and had continued there until 1998. He then moved to Apollo Hospital in New Delhi.

I still worked at the Batra hospital.

The kidney transplant programme continued at Batra Hospital throughout the next three decades with distinction – with two other senior surgeons joining the programme at Batra from AIIMS and the Army Hospital, New Delhi. The nephrology and kidney transplantation service of this hospital soon became a beacon of excellence, dedicated to care of patients and as an example of untiring teamwork in northern India.

When these two surgeons left, in 2014, an additional nephrologist and a kidney surgeon were appointed. The hospital-based Competent Authority was the body to approve related (grandmother, grandfather, mother, father, brother, sister, son, daughter, grandson and granddaughter above the age of eighteen years and spouse) transplant cases.

Though the Transplantation Act came into force in 1994 with modifications in later years, the clandestine transplant activities of paid unrelated kidney donors kept surfacing periodically across the country. This unlawful activity was generally carried out with fictitious documents and approvals obtained from inhouse hospital committees.

The whole story of the Kidney Scam at Batra Hospital is the story of an excellent undercover exercise in which the main players were the kingpin, let us call him O, and middlemen with associates spread all over the country. The hawk-eyes of the crime branch of the Delhi police and News24 TV channel together was what finally brought them down.

The sequence of events of this undercover operation was outlined by the Joint Commissioner of the Crime Branch of the Delhi Police after 40 days of surveillance and 200 hours of recorded evidence.

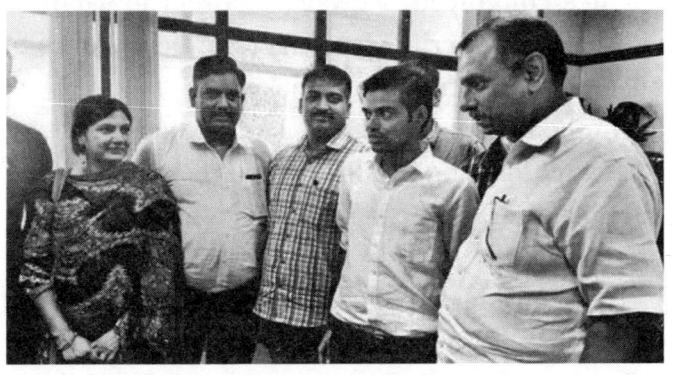

Decoy donor with police officials.

In April 2017, Jaideep, a young MBA student at Symbiosis College, Pune, originally from Rajasthan, had googled how to earn easy money by donating one of his kidneys after his friend, Rajesh, whom he had met in a coaching centre, had told him about the practice. Later, his anxiety and curiosity worsened when Rajesh went missing.

At this point, Jaideep decided to look deeper into the disappearance of his friend.

Jaideep got in touch with an agent whose whereabouts Rajesh had mentioned. He then decided to become a kidney donor himself and got in touch with the agent who introduced him to a kingpin, O, in Kolkata. The kingpin introduced him to one Rahul Sahu and a deal was struck. Thus, the illegal exercise of kidney donation was put into motion. Look at the reach of one single case – Pune, then Kolkata to Delhi and AP.

Jaideep was told by the touts to reach Delhi on a certain date. Upon reaching Delhi, the decoy donor approached News24 TV channel and was able to convince them about a pan-India kidney racket.

Once convinced, News24 channel journalists approached the crime branch of the Delhi Police to bust the kidney transplant racket.

On the 14th of April 2017, Jaideep had a meeting with a middleman in M-Block market in GK-I and later met the family of a kidney patient at Saket Mall on the same day.

The pimps had promised a sum of ₹4 lakh to the decoy donor, and a deal was done. The recipient, a rich person from Andhra Pradesh, had already been on biweekly hemodialysis in Batra Hospital for some time. All this occurred while the plain-clothed crime branch police personnel and News24 reporters were observing the proceedings of both meetings.

Jaideep was given a new identity – with a new name of Polepeddy Snayna Podma Phani Kumar – and was told to claim to be from Andhra Pradesh. He was made to learn Telugu and to become the 'second son' of the recipient, who had been a diabetic patient for 10 years. He also memorised the intricacies of living, language, food details, important family functions and happenings, the medical details of his 'new father', and the names of 'new siblings and mother'.

Jaideep underwent a complete makeover, from a haircut to his complexion, and was kept in an apartment in Hauz Rani with other potential donors. He was made to repeatedly recite his new name 'Polepeddy Snayna Podma Phani Kumar' and practiced writing and spelling his name correctly. He had to spend sufficient time with the family, who trained him to impersonate a Telugu accent. This incident shows how complicit with crime the families of recipients are. The rich completely lose sense of right and wrong.

The decoy donor was seen by the concerned senior nephrologist and transplant surgeon at Batra hospital and further specialised investigations as per transplant protocol were advised. He had invasive radiological investigations of kidney angiography to outline his kidney vessels and the ureter of his kidney.

To fully prove he was the recipient's son, a DNA test was performed at a city laboratory on the blood taken from the real son of the recipient under the name of the undercover donor to make it look like he was truly the biological son of the kidney recipient. Exhaustive details of documents and required investigations were performed under the direction of a medical team at Batra Hospital.

All original documents were changed to an identical profile in a well-crafted, fictitious manner. These included a birth certificate, SSC certificate, Aadhaar card, multiple photographs of the donor with the recipient and his family and siblings. All affidavits were created as per the Transplantation Act, including proof of substantial income of the donor and the recipient with false bank accounts, fake income tax return papers of the previous three years, a PAN card and a driving license. The racketeers even photoshopped pictures of the recipient's real son so that the donor resembled him.

The donor, Jaideep, underwent intensive coaching and counseling in preparation to present himself to the internal competent authority. It had included details of the family to make him look like the 'real son' of the recipient, Mr Polepeddy Venkata Ramana and his 'mother' Mrs P Nacharamma, along with his 'elder brother', Mr P Kartick P Kumar. Jaideep was made to memorise the names of his fictitious grandparents, Mr P Nacharamma and Mrs P Padmavati.

A psychiatric evaluation of the donor was also performed at the hospital to make sure he was fit for donation in every way. It all appears to be a well-conceived and meticulously executed makeover exercise by all involved in this dangerous saga of 'unrelated transplant' for approval by the Internal Competent Authority and bypass the Hospital-based Authorisation Committee for Transplantation, which includes government-appointed essential members from outside the hospital.

Jaideep was explicitly briefed on all the details of the meeting of the internal authorisation committee and was told the questions that would be asked by the panel. He was thoroughly tutored to identify all the documents submitted in his name. In the meeting, the decoy donor deliberately answered some questions incorrectly as he was going along with all the steps covered so far.

It appeared that members of the committee confined themselves to scrutiny of submitted documents, and he was not scrutinised or questioned to determine the authenticity of his presented profile. An inhouse approval for transplantation was granted.

Since the concerned consultant nephrologist was on leave for two weeks, the date of transplantation was deferred from the 14th of April to the 23rd May, and this intervening period was ample time to prepare for this horrid exercise. Since the members of the entire gang were operating from different parts of northern India and Kolkata, they had enough time to reach New Delhi in time on the 22nd May 2017.

The gang kingpin in Kolkata was the person who had referred the Hyderabad-based family looking for a donor to his accomplice in Delhi. This kingpin had been in regular contact with his counterparts in Hyderabad and elsewhere in the country.

The 32-year-old accomplice was assigned to do field work in Delhi; he was the first contact for undercover donors, and he arranged the meetings with the recipient family.

A 27-year-old female member of the gang was responsible for counseling and liaison work for this decoy donor and other real prospective donors in an apartment at Hauz Rani.

The fourth member of the group, who was 45 years old, prepared the forged documents and kept frequent and close contact with concerned hospital members. Another 33-year-old member of the gang was responsible for taking care of the donors.

The crime branch was in possession of 200 hours of recorded video, and both – the reporter from the News24 TV channel and the decoy donor – had been given spy devices for their 40 days of surveillance.

Two gang members were arrested the night before the date of the transplantation. They disclosed that a sum of ₹30 lakh had already been collected by the Delhi accomplice from the recipient, and the decoy donor had not been paid any amount at that stage.

The crime branch of the Delhi police swung into action on the morning of 25 May, the day of the kidney transplantation, and raided Batra Hospital. The decoy donor was taken away from the hospital along with all relevant documents.

All this undercover action took place right under my nose without I or anyone else in the department getting to know about the presence of the police and the media.

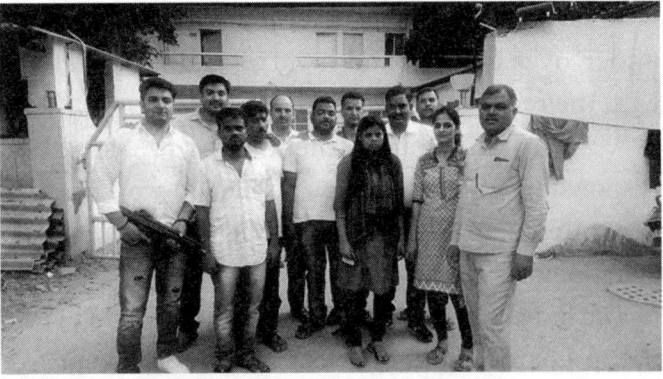

Four people, including a woman, arrested by Crime Branch of Delhi Police. Photo is from *The Indian Express* website and newspaper.

While the final 'act of transplantation' was in progress in Batra Hospital, a thrilling 'cat-and-mouse chase' was in progress between a middleman of the racket and a sub-inspector on a south Delhi road. She was assigned to keep an eye on two suspected middlemen who were staying at the guest house in Hauz Rani. The other members of the crime branch police were reaching Batra Hospital where the decoy donor was admitted for transplantation. A few minutes before the raid, the sub-inspector sighted two suspects leaving the guest house in separate cars. She, in her personal car and accompanied by a tea-seller working in her office, drove several kilometers behind the two cars of the suspects, which took different routes.

She chose to continue chasing a man known as Rahul, the alleged tout, who soon realised that he was being followed and made sudden turns and u-turns on the road. Ultimately, he decided to stop his car and to confront the lady driver. She lied and told him that her friend, the tea seller, bet her that she couldn't trail him for 60 kilometers, so she was trying to prove him wrong. Rahul was not convinced and wanted to get away quickly.

Subsequently, the lady sub-inspector needed to keep him in sight until help from her colleagues arrived, so she invited him for a cup of coffee at a shop in Kishangarh, in the Vasant Kunj area. The unwilling Rahul obliged, but ordered only soft drinks, as he wanted to finish quickly and leave. To delay his departure, she ordered herself a large cup of coffee and was able to engage him in conversation, while she secretly dialed her crime branch colleagues. She was deliberately talking in a loud voice, describing the locality and circumstances she was in, and a nearby policeman was smart enough to take the hint and quickly send a police team to the café. This is how alias Rahul was arrested on the spot.

The crime branch of the Delhi police interrupted the transplantation on 25 May 2017, and the prospective donor was taken away for interrogation by them.

A few outside persons (the middlemen) had already been apprehended by Delhi police. There was continuous coverage of the event on TV channels and print media for a week by News24 and others. There were live interviews of chosen personnel from the Directorate General of Health Services, officials from the Government of Delhi and Delhi Medical Council, including with Deputy Chief Minister Manish Sisodia.

It took the crime branch six months to complete all of the investigations. There were interrogative meetings called by the Health and Family Welfare Department of the Government of Delhi. Batra Hospital's transplantation license was suspended. Simultaneously, the HLA matching work done at a prominent laboratory in Delhi was also suspended for three months by the Government of Delhi.

RECOMMENCING KIDNEY TRANSPLANTATION AT BATRA HOSPITAL

Re-inspection of the nephrology and transplantation department at Batra Hospital by a committee constituted by the Delhi Organ Transplant Cell was done on 17 January 2018, after the hospital put in place a new transplant surgeon and a new nephrologist.

The hospital was then permitted to reopen the department and commence transplants, once again in June 2018. Resumption letter for renal transplantation was received by the hospital on 9 March 2018. By then, a sizable number of patients waiting for transplantation had been moved to other centres. One patient reportedly lost her life in the hands of someone again called 'Dr Amit Kumar'. Another patient died with chest complications when waiting for transplantation.

The footfall of new patients at Batra became practically zero, and it was presumed that kidney transplantation had been discontinued at Batra Hospital permanently. In such an adverse environment, resuming transplantation was a difficult task, and one had to wait for an ideal recipient and donor for transplantation work to begin again. As the chief nephrologist of the department, the onus of this arduous task fell on me.

A young medical student had consulted the author with problems of high blood pressure and early kidney failure one year before the scandal, and over a period of time, his kidney function had deteriorated.

His family was apprised of the urgent need of a kidney transplant, and his mother was of a similar blood group. Both mother and son were admitted to Batra Hospital on 28th May 2018 in the nephrology ward. The transplant date was tentatively scheduled for a Monday next week.

The patient was started on hemodialysis on his second day of admission and treatment was modified. In his case, all investigations of transplantation were completed in three days.

A detailed battery of investigations of the mother were undertaken with precision, as per protocol. An isotope scan, which was used to prove that both her kidneys were working simultaneously, could not be done in the hospital for some reasons and instead was done at the National Heart Hospital. The report was obtained instantly, saying she had been cleared to be a donor for her son.

The HLA and DR Tissue typing could not be done at the previous lab, as their contract to work for Batra hospital had been terminated.

A new contract with Ranbaxy Laboratories was made in an hour, surmounting all hurdles of the various departments involved. The paperwork and a video camera recording of the blood collection in the presence of the hospital's laboratory in-charge, the transplant coordinator and a representative of the Ranbaxy Lab, were done against time.

On the same day, the donor underwent CT renal angiography, a psychiatric evaluation, and a gynecological examination.

The surgical team was informed and after detailed examination of the recipient and the donor, a complete scrutiny of documents as per the Transplant Act was undertaken by the entire team involved.

The hospital's competent authority was then informed. The relevant documents' file was handed over to the Deputy Medical Superintendent – Transplant Cell of the hospital.

The competent authority meeting was convened on the following Saturday morning at 11 am, with all new members, who were constituted after the resumption letter was received.

This meeting lasted for over an hour, and one member of the committee opined that the committee was *not empowered* to approve *this* case.

The transplant coordinator told the committee that no provision for related transplantation (mother and son) was applicable as per the Act. The approval was then signed with a rider to obtain the 'HLA typing report' before transplantation was carried out on Monday morning.

The colour doppler study of pelvic vessels was performed on Sunday and SRL Laboratory (the Ranbaxy lab) issued the HLA report and it was crossmatched at 8 a.m. on Monday. The transplantation was performed without any problem.

The donor was discharged on the 5th day after transplantation, and the recipient left the hospital on the 11th day.

Thus, kidney transplantation at Batra Hospital was successfully restarted after a full year.[4]

---

[4] References: https://medicaldialogues.in – 27.5.17,
https://m.dailyhunt.in – 25.5.17,
https://www.dnaindia.com – 28.5.17,

THE ARMY RESEARCH AND REFERRAL HOSPITAL

The Times of India, New Delhi
Wednesday, October 13, 2004

TIMES CITY

Kidney scam: Army hospital asked to submit relevant documents

Even this prestigious institution has not been spared allegations of transplanting traded kidneys.

A native of Bihar called Kishan had filed a complaint in February 2004 with the Delhi Police that one of his kidneys was removed at the Army Research and Referral Hospital – without his consent.

Kishan had told the police, he was taken by three accomplices – namely SS, Raj and VKP (names changed) to the Army Hospital in Delhi. They had taken him to this hospital for backache and on returning to his home, a reexamination had revealed that his left kidney was not present and was allegedly removed for kidney transplantation.

A city court had demanded presentation of all original documents for verification and scrutiny

KIDNEY SCAMS IN DELHI

https://www.hindustantimes.com – 1.6.17,
https://www.hindustantimes.com – 2.7.17,
https://www.dnaindia.com – 28.5.17,
https://in.news – 26.5.17,
https://www.dailypioneer.com – 27.5.17,
https://www.newindianexpress.com – 1.6.17,
https://odishasuntimes.com – 26.5.17,
https://www.dnaindia.com – 27.5.17,
https://www.hindustantimes.com – 2.7.17,
https://indianexpress.com – 27.5.17,
https://www.hindustantimes.com – 1.6.17,
https://www.jagran.com – 28.5.17,
https://www.hindustantimes.com – 27.5.17.

by a committee of experts. It was reported that an internal enquiry had already been in action. The fate of internal committee of the hospital and further developments in court proceedings, as usual, is not available to the public. Because the hospital is for army personnel, a shroud of secrecy envelopes this straight-forward case of crime even now, almost fifteen years later.

VIP AND FAST-TRACK KIDNEY TRANSPLANTATION

The first high-profile VIP case in a Delhi hospital was that of Loknayak Jayaprakash Narayan in the late '70s.

In India, kidney transplantation for all is available and practiced in hospitals across the country.

In the eighties and nineties, the rich and well-to-do patients went abroad for kidney transplantation, with donors taken from their home country, India.

Notably in the recent past, two VIP and fast-tracked kidney transplantations took place in the capital of the nation at AIIMS, New Delhi. The kidney transplantation of the foreign minister and the finance minister of the Union Cabinet in the Government of India were undertaken in 2018.

According to AIIMS sources, for Sushma Swarajji, the kidney was donated by a woman in her forties, not related to the Foreign Minister. The print media has published all kinds of details, and it is said that a distant relative, legally classified as an 'unrelated donor' whose blood group matched, had agreed to donate a kidney to the then Foreign Minister. It is said that the Minister got clearance for her surgery 'in a matter of days'.

Hospital authorities had at the time clarified that the operation was not planned in the list of operations, and requisite paperwork was done through regular channels, and all guidelines prescribed in the Act were strictly followed.[5]

The second VIP transplant was in the case of the union cabinet's Finance Minister, Arun Jaitleyji which also took place at AIIMS. His kidney was donated by a distant relative, a middle-aged woman in the category of 'living unrelated donation', and the authorisation committee had given its approval after all documentation was completed. It is said that his transplantation also was on a fast-track basis as his condition was rather unstable and carried out under a prescribed clause of the Act.[6]

---

[5] References: The Transplantation of Human Organs and Tissues Act, 1994 with The Transplantation of Human Organs and Tissues Rules, 2014;
http://indianexpress.com/article/india/sushma-swarajs-kidney-transplant-at-aiims – 10.12.16;
http://scroll.in/pulse/824175/sushma-swarajs-kidney-transplant – 15.12.16.
[6] http://www.ndtv.com/india-news/arun-jaitley-undergoes-kidney-transplant – 14.5.18; *The Indian Express* – 14.5.18.

CYBER SCAMS IN KIDNEY TRADE

OF ALL KIDNEY SCAMS, THE cyber scams are the most dangerous. They are invisible, 'uniformly fake' and hundreds and thousands of money transfers take place online to unknown and fraudulent entities without any gain to the donor and often, to the recipient, leading to disaster in a desperate situation when a patient has identified a suitable kidney for himself and is unable to benefit from it.

For the international kidney trade, the internet is a powerful tool and is widely used by all in the world. Successful outcome is extremely doubtful and the cyber trading of organs is an organised crime. The trading of organs is a multi-level, fast moving crime in which a desperate seller, middlemen, hospital staff, doctors, buyers and in some cases organ banks are involved.

In a majority of the cases, swindlers, traffickers, the gullible and illiterate individuals are victims. The fake advertisements of 'kidney sale, kidney available, kidneys for a price' and fake foundation for organ donation and similar websites proclaiming and advertising these are all part of a large-scale internet scam.

There are donors selling their kidneys with attractive details and deals are frequently struck remotely, with the faces of not only the donor and recipient unseen, but the kingpin, touts, all unknown, unseen. The countries where internet trade of organs is prevalent include South Africa, Nigeria and in other African countries. In India, however, where the trade is most alive and prosperous, there is no soliciting of kidneys like grooms and brides on websites.

African cyber criminals posing as doctors offering to pay up to $130,000 to buy live kidneys, as part of a ploy to extract personal and bank account details from gullible victims, have been targeting Dubai in recent months and medical and internet experts have warned online users to be vigilant of the scams.

In India, fake hospital websites are aplenty and in Delhi alone there are such websites of all major hospitals such as Apollo Hospital, Batra Hospital, Medanta Hospital, Fortis Hospital, Max Hospital and others.

An example of a kidney sale offer on the internet goes like this:

> South Africa X: Hi, I'm a healthy white South African in desperate need of financial aid. Is there any way I can do this from South Africa? Sell my kidney that is.
>
> Unknown Y: Hello. The above is my e-mail. I'm in South Africa. Young, healthy and white. I'm in desperate need of money. What can I get for my kidney and is it safe?

Amir from Nepal writes: I was selling it for @3500 to save my car going back to the bank. A lot of people contacted [and] me, asked for [a] free kidney. Some wanted me to come to India. A lot of people from Dubai called. Mostly brokers contacted me.

Name Z: Age 23   Muslim
No Kidney Problem With The Grace Of ALLAH
                                                     No Drink
Blood Group AB+   No Smoke Never   Weight 78 Kg
Height 5.9   Country Pakistan   City Peshawar
Qualification BBA (HONS) From Peshawar University.

INTERNET FRAUD IN KOLKATA – NIGERIAN INVOLVED

In 2017, a 32-year-old Nigerian man, David Ujma Uba, was arrested by the police in India for allegedly running a massive kidney donation scam in which he defrauded over 10 people of ₹3 crore (about N16.55 million).

In the *Times of India* it was reported that Uba, who arrived in the country on a tourist visa in 2013 from Nigeria, had created a fake hospital website and ran advertisements in some national papers where he promised to help his victims secure donated kidneys. Uba was said to have asked anyone in need of a kidney to contact him as he had a 'bank of kidneys' to sell.

A police statement said Uba asked those who contacted him to pay various sums into his bank account but failed to render the services he had advertised and when they realised they had been scammed, a victim filed a complaint with the Kolkata Cyber Crime Police in April 2017.

BANGALORE – WHATSAPP AD KIDNEY SALE

Man falls for WhatsApp ad and tries to sell kidney for Rs 1.6 crore. This is what happened next

In this fraud in a WhatsApp message, the Head of Renal Transplant Surgery at Columbia Asia Hospital in Bangalore, was impersonated. Someone had tried to con a person called S Shekhar (name changed) who was in dire need of money and had been assured a sum of ₹1.6 crore for his kidney.

This gentleman, Shekhar, came to the said hospital and showed the hospital authorities all the WhatsApp messages and subsequent conversations he had had with a recipient representative on various dates (this was with the impersonator actually).

The hospital filed a complaint with the cyber police and it had registered a case under section 66(C) and 66(D) of the Information Technology Act of 2000 and 120B (criminal conspiracy) 468 (forgery for purpose of cheating), 420 (cheating), 471 (using as genuine a forged document) of the Indian Penal Code (IPC) along with other sections of the IPC. Follow up details are not known.

ANDHRA PRADESH – ONLINE KIDNEY RACKET

In November 2018, Mehboob Nagar police arrested a man called SHS (name changed), 44, from Guntakal in Anantapur district of Andhra Pradesh. He worked as a petty rice trader and had posed as a kidney doctor. He called himself Dr Anand.

Through various messages on social networking sites, Anand promised to pay up to ₹50 lakh each to kidney donors.

When a prospective recipient contacted him on the phone, he was made to deposit ₹10,000 first as a fee in a bank account and as soon as the money was deposited, Dr Anand's mobile phone would stop responding to phone calls of the victims. He managed to get his friend's identity cards, with which as proof he had opened an account in Axis Bank in the name of Kumnari Gussapa. One of his victims called Kiran had decided to go to the hometown of this impersonator and helped police to arrest him.

FACEBOOK KIDNEY RACKET

There have been some feeble attempts to solicit recipients for a kidney on the Facebook. It has not become a regular practice at this stage.

In May 2014, a high-ranking IPS official in the rank of Inspector General of Police (Civil Defense), had filed a complaint with the local police in Lucknow that a gang was in communication on Facebook with offers of ₹3.5 lakh to ₹4 lakh for a kidney. The IG had himself offered to sell one of his kidneys and was asked if he possessed a passport and should visit Pune and he was told that he would be taken for a trip abroad. The fate of this particular complaint five years ago is also not known.

There are a large number of fake websites, however:

Whatsapp and call: +916385533074
Email: drthachiljoseph@apollohospitalwideworld.com (//apollohospitalwideworl.com)
Email at: Apollohospital.rao@gmail.com (//gmail.com)
Email us: drwesleydavid@colombiaasiahospital.com (//colombiaasiahospital.com)
Whatsapp at: +916385533076
Email: drthachiljoseph@apollohospitalwideworld.com (//apollohospitalwideworld.com)
Call and whatsapp on: +916385533074
Get money 4cr, we need donor very urgent (Bangalore, India)

Posting date: 30 November 2018.

Attention plz, if you need in money or you want money urgent, contact us immediately 9958820908, you can whatsapp us on 9958820908. If you want solve your all financial problem, than don't delay contact us immediately 9958820908.

CYBER SCAMS IN KIDNEY TRADE

(This ad is relevant for Bangalore: Get money 4 cr. We need donor very urgent Health Medical, Bangalore, India.)

Posting date: 30 November 2018.

Donate Kidney for 3 cr in Apollo Hospital, Bangalore, India.

Hi, were looking for kidney donors in Apollo Hospital, very urgently. B plus +ve, O plus +ve, O plus and A plus +ve with valid Id proof for the amount of 3,00,00,000.00 Crore Rupees contact whatsapp Plus 917838938108 or call for more information.

(This ad is relevant for Bangalore: Donate kidney for 3 CR in Apollo Hospital Health Medical, Bangalore, India.)

Posting date: 3 November 2018

Hello (Patna, India)

Hello, are you interested to selling one of your thesaurus (sic.) for a good amount of {2 crore} in India pls kindly contact us now Reply below as were looking for Thesaurus donor, Very urgently who are group B, group A, O plus +ve and O plus +ve. Interested donor should contact us now. Best regards plus 919751213754.

(This ad is relevant for – Patna Hello Sale Business – Patna, India.)

I want to sell my kidney for money contact us (Visakhapatnam, India).

Hello everyone, we urgently needed A, B, O blood group donors between the age of 18–60. We give you all the entire best attempt, we will give you honest price of 1 CR, 50 LAKS india money best treatment for your transplant as top best medical treatment it will help your future life, kindly contact us on whatsapp plus 918296067169 for more infor...

Vishakhapatnam: I want sell my kidney for money contact us Beauty Care – Visakhaptnam, India.

(This ad is relevant for – Visakhapatnam.)

Give one kidney and be rewarded with 3,00,00,000.00 Crore rupees as we need Organ donor urgently in

Apollo Hospital for patients who face life time dialysis problem unless they under go kidney transplant. Contact Whatsapp or Call 917838938108, Whatsapp plus 917838938108.

(This ad is relevant for – Visakhapatnam Freedom for All contact for 3 Crore Beauty Care – Visakhapatnam, India.)[1]

Posting date: 30 November 2018.

How to sell ur kidney and how much you can get (Visakhapatnam, India).

Are you interested to selling one of your kidney for a good amount of 4 Crore {Advance money 2 Crore} in India pls kindly contact us now on our email as we are looking for kidney donor, Very urgently who are group B, group A, O +ve and O +ve. Interested person should contact us Dr Chetan Shah. Call number Plus 917066658255 Whatsapp Plus 917066658255.

FAKE WHATSAPP MESSAGE LINKS MUMBAI DOCTOR TO KIDNEY RACKET

Internet is inundated with fake websites and advertisements of either selling a kidney or buying a kidney with attractive offers to both gullible donors and recipient at par. In this worldwide 'fake kidney bazaar' there are no kidneys available and sizable amount of money disappears in each misadventure and it cannot be retrieved.

[1] https://www.thehindu.com/news/national/andhra-pradesh/kidneyracket-report-to-be-ready-in-a-week/ article27105710.ece

KIDNEY RACKETS WORLDWIDE

FOR MANY DECADES, ILLEGAL ORGAN trade has been reported across the world. From early nineties to present date, most cases have been reported from African countries, Middle East, Pakistan, Sri Lanka, Bangladesh and Nepal.

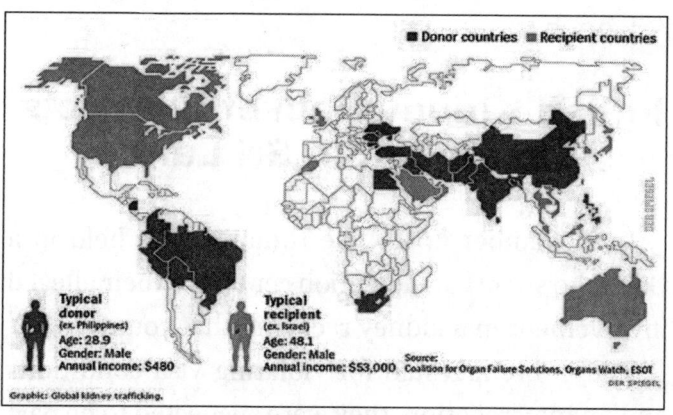

The Kidney World Order.

In 2018, five Nepali nationals were arrested for allegedly persuading villagers to sell their kidneys, who they smuggled into India. Most scams here come to light in the border district of Chitwan. Chitwan district police arrested the accused from Chitwan, Kathmandu and Rasuwa districts, the Deputy Superintendent of Police (DSP) reported.

They targeted gullible villagers and took them in confidence with fake promises before extracting their kidneys and they send the prospective donors to various hospitals in India. 'They used to charge a commission of ₹50,000 to ₹100,000 for finding people willing to sell their kidney in exchange of monetary gains and establishing their contact with smugglers', the police in Nepal said.

The Chitwan police has now formed a seven-member Medical Response Team (MRT) to look into crimes related to health, following which this racket was busted. The accused will be charged under the Human Trafficking and Transportation (Control) Act, 2007.[1]

Indian Kidney Racket Suspects Remanded In Sri Lanka

In November 2016, five Indians were held in a Colombo suburban detention centre for their alleged involvement in a kidney racket in that country.

They were arrested for violating visa conditions and on interrogation, they were suspected to be part of a kidney racket in that country. The police in Sri Lanka had intensive exchange of information with

[1] https://www.ndtv.com – 30.7.18.

the Indian police and six doctors said they suspected six Sri Lankan doctors of involvement in the illegal kidney transplantation. The kidney transplantation of foreign national's kidney was prohibited in Sri Lanka in January 2016.[2]

In July 2018, Mumbai police investigated an international kidney racket in which an Indian recipient and donor both were involved in surgeries done in Cairo, Egypt. The kingpin, let us call him P, was a well-known middleman in Ahmedabad and the donors were lured from poor families in Mumbai and were flown to Egypt.

VISA BOMB IN EGYPT

In another case, an impoverished 29-year-old man from his native village Taloga, in Vellore in Tamil Nadu, was lured into a driver's job in Cairo. He had migrated to Mumbai in 2014 and was driving aggregator cabs and was unable to make his ends meet.

The Vellore man had contacted an Ahmedabad-based *shiksha consultancy* for a job abroad. This consultancy was run by the racket's mastermind and the job seeker travelled in June to Ahmedabad, where he underwent certain blood investigations. On 15 July, he was sent to Cairo.

In Cairo, he was taken to an apartment where five other people were staying. The very next day, he was taken to the Nile Badrawi Hospital for blood

---

[2] Reference: https://www.ndtv.com – 12.11.16,
https://www.jagran.com – 23.1.16.

tests and scans and was taken to the Indian embassy, local police station and health offices and was made to sign Arabic papers. Once the formalities were complete, the 'visa bomb' was dropped – that his 15-day visa was to expire and his only option to leave Cairo officially was to donate a kidney, otherwise he would languish in a Cairo jail. Simultaneously, the driver was offered ₹2,000,000 and, therefore, the man from Vellore had agreed to 'donate' the kidney under coercion.

> **'Donate your kidney or face jail in Cairo'**
>
> Mumbai The Sahar Police investigating the alleged international kidney racket said most recipients and donors are Indians. They said the surgeries performed on four of the six Indians, to harvest their kidneys, were done in Cairo, Egypt. The police wants to make the donors as witnesses. They said all the donors are poor and hail from states such as Kerala, Andhra Pradesh and Jammu and Kashmir.
>
> Cops said Nizam lured donors from poor families and sent them to Egypt with Prajapati's help, who arranged for passports, tickets and visas. The donors were flown to Egypt via Mumbai and Delhi. While the donors were paid Rs5 lakh, the duo took much more from the recipients.
>
> https://www.hindustantimes.com/mumbai-news/international-kidney-racket-mumbai-cops-say-most-donors-recipients-are-indians/story-UayRQgEcds1...

BONDED LABOUR IN PAKISTAN

The 21st century saw an increased number of international visitors to Pakistan for organ transplantation. This trade flourished from the time the organ transplantation act was promulgated in neighbour India. A large number of Indian patients made a bee line for kidney transplantation in Pakistan with kidneys obtained from the impoverished Pakistani population.

Pakistan promulgated the 'Transplantation of Human Organs and Tissues Ordinance (THOTO)' in September 2007. In this legislation, a crucial clause was 'donation by Pakistani citizens shall not be permissible to citizens of other countries'. Any person found to be in violation of this or involved in any commercial organ dealings is subject to 10 years imprisonment and a fine of 1,000,000 Pak rupees.

Following this ordinance, like in India, the number of the transplants from unrelated donors gradually increased in Pakistan and patients from countries from the middle east received paid kidneys in private clinics in Pakistan. Two private hospitals in Lahore and Rawalpindi were involved in carrying out transplants surreptitiously for non-Pakistani citizens. At present, there is considerable resistance among the Pakistani public against donation of organs following death due to religious compulsions and the trade and trafficking in organs is still prevalent.[3]

Pakistani kidneys attracting foreigners

LAHORE: An increased number of visitors from abroad are travelling to the country to fly out with a brand new kidney, and Pakistan is now thought to be a growing centre of global 'organ tourism'. The trade has flourished in the country, most notably since India placed a ban on the practice 10 years ago, diverting traffic to Pakistan.

"It is spurred on by the desperate poverty of people, by the lack of laws and by unscrupulous doctors, clinics and their 'agents'," said Dr Yasir Agha, a urologist who has recently begun practice in Lahore. Idrees, 27, is a free man, after nearly 10 years in bondage at a brick-kiln near Sheikhupura, 100 kilometre north of Lahore.

He won his freedom by selling his left kidney. With the Rs 90,000 he got, he was able to pay off a debt of around Rs 60,000 he and his elderly parents owed to the kiln owner. The debt had accumulated over nearly 15 years. But after paying off the amount, he had little left over, and less than six months after undergoing surgery at a private clinic to remove his kidney, he is once more in debt, having borrowed Rs 5,000 from a cousin a few days ago.

"It's a pity I can't sell my other kidney," he said only half jokingly, adding: "But at least we are free. Allah will help us now." Though debt bondage is banned under the 1992 Bonded Labour Abolition Act, it flourishes at kilns scattered across the central Punjab province and on agricultural estates in the southern province of Sindh.

"The continued existence of bonded labour shows that the authorities simply have no wish to see it end or to enforce the law," Asma Jahangir, a leading lawyer, rights activist and HRCP chairperson, told IRIN.

She added: "We will just have to fight on for the rights of people enslaved by debt." An appeal, seeking the upholding of the law on bonded labour, is now before the Supreme Court. It was moved by the HRCP after the Sindh High Court in 2002 dismissed the petitions of 94 bonded farm workers, and ruled that disputes over debt should be settled under the Sindh Tenancy Act of 1950. HRCP pointed out that the Sindh High Court had failed to make any reference to the 1992 law banning debt bondage. IRIN

---

[3] References: *Daily Times,* Lahore, Safar 29, 1426 (April 9, 2005) Pakistan's kidney trade: An overview Vol.62, No.1, January 2012, J Pak Med Assoc; Pakistan a haven for human organs trade: chief justice (internet). *Indo Asian News Service.* 2007 Jul 26.

DEATH ROW PRISONERS IN ASIA

The organs of executed prisoners are being used for transplant operations in Taiwan despite much controversy. The death penalty is given for a range of crimes in Taiwan, including murder, rape, kidnapping, and sedition. Since October 1990, when organ transplantation from executed prisoners began, there have been 51 executions and 22 prisoners have donated organs. Execution is normally carried out by shooting through the heart, but when a prisoner consents to organ donation, execution is by a shot to the head.

In the early nineties, Hong Kong Hospital had an established practice of transplant of kidney harvested from prisoners executed in mainland China.

Authorities in Hong Kong said, the organs were obtained with prior consent of prisoners and their families. Middlemen and brokers were charging as much as $30,000 to obtain a kidney from China.

Executions are still very common in China and death penalty is applied for a wide range of crimes, from murder, rape and robbery, to smuggling, embezzlement and bribery. The number of executions is thought to run to several thousand a year.

The Chinese Medical Association, a member of the World Medical Association, is reluctant to comment on the issue, and a spokeswoman described the practice as a 'matter of personal choice'.

IN SOUTH AMERICA

Evidence of the trafficking of human organs, the murder of patients and fraud was uncovered by an

Argentine judicial investigation into irregularities at a state-run mental institution in the city of Lujan, just outside Buenos Aires a few years ago.

As a result of testimonies from health workers, bodies of former patients were exhumed and it was found that their corneas and other organs had been harvested and sold and blood was drained for storage in a blood bank.[4]

Argentina uncovers patients killed for organs

As a result of testimonies from health workers, bodies of former patients have been exhumed. Government investigators claim that corneas and other organs were sold by Dr Sanchez and his accomplices and that patients' blood was drained for storage in the blood bank of his own private clinic.

[4] BMJ Volume-204, 25 April 1992.

THE HUMAN ELEMENT

ROLE OF THE MEDIA

THE MEDIA IN THE SEVENTIES and eighties published colourful and sensational news regarding kidney racketeering in India. These publications may have had some positive effect in highlighting the trade. But it is also possible that the widespread publicity actually perpetuated the 'kidney rackets' as many more people got to know of the possibility a healthy kidney offered.

The media had their share in making India a 'kidney bazaar', where one could buy a kidney at the cheapest price and get away with it by giving wide publicity to the process.

Saheb, the Anil Kapoor and Amrita Singh film about a football player who sells one of his kidneys in order to get dowry to marry off his sister, is just a small example of how organ transplant used to be portrayed negatively in India not so long ago. Even many 'related' donors have backed out after seeing the film, and there were multiple negative programmes which did not paint a healthy picture of kidney transplantations or any organ donation at all.

The exception is *Bucket List,* a 2018 Indian Marathi language comedy-drama film featuring Madhuri Dixit where a heart donation is shown in a positive and glamourous light.

An Australian TV programme 'Kidney Agents' showed prisoners in the Philippines, Malaysia and Thailand offering their organs to agents who were in league with prison authorities. Germans were said to 'import' live donors from east Europe. Even in London, transplant clinics had passed off live 'unrelated' donors as 'relatives' of the patients.

One must remember, organ donation is not a crime and organs are needed to save lives. It has to be, however, done legally, within the ambit of Indian laws and overboard with real documentation. The media has a great role to play in increasing awareness about organ transplants and donations.

CHANGED PATTERN OF KIDNEY TRADE

Since the late nineties, till today, organ trade scams and scandals in India have evolved into identity theft, coercion and deceit, false promises and gruesome exploitation of uneducated and oppressed people.

The rich have taken impoverished donors for kidney transplantation to neighbouring countries like Sri Lanka, Turkey and Singapore. Since India is a large country, such donors are even taken from northern India to hospitals in the south of the country.

Alternatively, for a recipient, fake documents and family photographs with prospective donor are submitted to the regional transplant authorisation committees for approval. With all formalities of documentation complete, the unrelated donor is counseled for authentication of familiarity with recipient, and the recipient and their family are tutored for veracity of all aspects of presentation before the authorisation committee. This elaborate exercise has a multi-layered support system of touts, middlemen and powerful gang leaders forming a syndicate in the kidney trade.

The provisions of punishment for commercialism are quite elaborate in terms of every aspect of procuring a kidney by any means and maximum penalties of imprisonment of 5 to 10 years and a fine ranging between ₹20 lakh to ₹100 lakh. However, usually, in every State of India – the investigations remain incomplete at every level.

The role of doctors and hospitals have always been doubted and police and local courts have often indicted and penalised with suspension of services. However, very rarely are fines and imprisonments awarded. The participation of hospitals and their employees – and their collusion with convicted middlemen and members of their teams under trail – continue unchecked in their status quo mode for many many years and the course of justice is almost never completed.

Human beings, like all living things, are basically domineering.

In the history of civilisation, behavioural studies of animals, insects and plants document the 'dominance factor' and aggressive behaviour of mankind appears to be intrinsic. Man, in his existence of 1.4 million years, is known to acquire power *at any cost*. With the rapid advancement of technology, the aggression in Man has become more unscrupulous, virulent and destructive. Subjugation and exploitation of the less privileged has always been the norm throughout the history of civilisation, and this practice has been prevalent in many societies throughout time – as examples can be cited the slave trades of the Roman empire, the slave trades of the West in the 17th, 18th and 19th centuries, migration scams and organ trades of the 21st century.

The instances of fraud, misappropriation of wealth and corruption scams are worldwide and human trafficking in less-economically developed countries is rampant. The poorest of the poor get trapped easily and with prevalent gender bias, females are more vulnerable in less developed countries. Women are often forced under emotional, social and financial burdens of a family, to surrender to violence, including being sold as kidney donors by husbands and families.

SON OVER DAUGHTER

Gender bias is so severe in Indian society that even mothers are violent to the girl child, it has to be experienced to be believed.

I recall an incident from the 1990s, where two children – a brother and sister – were brought for hospital care. The boy and girl were both brought with polycystic kidneys. It is an inherited condition where the children are born with multiple cysts in their kidneys.

Two decades later the family came back to the hospital. The 23-year-old unmarried daughter had grossly abnormal kidney functioning. She came in with great swelling of her body and hemodialysis was started at once for her. Both the parents came with apparently equal concern for the daughter.

We advised the family that the young patient was in urgent need of a kidney transplant. Both parents had similar blood groups. The mother showed initial eagerness to donate. However, her kidneys matched imperfectly. So, it was the father who became the prospective donor.

The father was medically examined for compatibility. A date was finally fixed for the transplant. At this point, the mother, who was responsible for both the donor and the recipient in the family, developed cold feet. We do not have any information actually as to what happened. The mother, as next of kin, refused to do the formalities needed for a transplant under the Transplant Act. The family soon checked out of the hospital.

The young woman came for hemodialysis sporadically, as an outpatient. We did not know for quite some time how her care progressed. Until one day, the young woman was brought to hospital unconscious and gasping for breath. Of course, her kidneys were failing and a few days later, she died.

There was no sign of grief on the mother's face. The daughter was unmarried and a financial liability. So, the mother, by neglect, simply let the daughter die.

A few months later, the son too was brought to the hospital with gross kidney failure. He too urgently needed a kidney transplant. This time, the mother readily came forward to be a kidney donor and the young man lived with a transplant done from the mother.

This was a painful truth that we doctors and nurses at the hospital had to reconcile to and live with. It is India's reality – a boy, no matter how ill, preferred over a girl, equally unwell.

India, with its population of 1.3 billion – is a vast and heterogeneous country. Scandals and scams are inevitable. But after fifty years in the profession, I have a question. Must this country continue to be the Mecca of the live kidney trade? There are stringent laws now, the living standard of Indians has improved considerably, says the government. We have some data on annual accident deaths and other kinds of deaths in the country, we have the beginning of a registry of annual kidney transplants happening and a rough estimate of what is needed. India's medical fraternity is renowned worldwide and its judiciary and vibrant media are well known for championing legitimate causes and helping the underprivileged. Still, can nothing be done to change India's profile as the world's biggest kidney bazaar?

MOVING FORWARD

INDIA'S IDEAL UNRELATED KIDNEY DONOR

INDIA HAS THE LARGEST NUMBER of traffic accidents in the world.

While Chennai records most road traffic accidents, the highest number of fatal accidents have been recorded in Delhi, according to a Transport Ministry report of 2016. This report said, the number of road traffic accidents in Tamil Nadu was 71,431 the previous year whereas total number of deaths was 150,000 in the deadly roads of this country. It amounts to 55 accidents per hour and 17 deaths in 60 minutes on Indian roads every day. The large population of 1.3 billion people, high density of traffic, extremely poor conditions of road and inadequate traffic management all contribute to this dismal state of affairs.

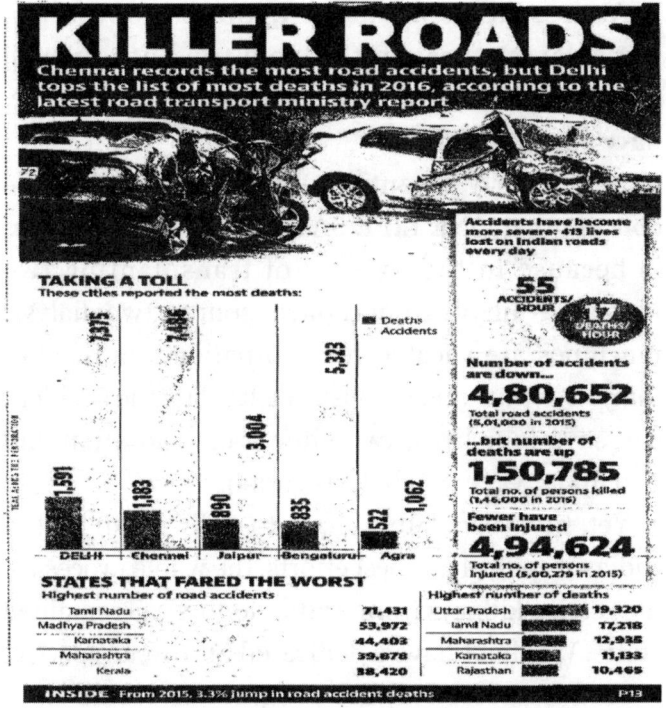

It is a pity that we are unable to harvest the organs of people dying on our roads. This is primarily because of immediately unavailable skilled personnel and storage facilities at accident sites and the delays that occur in transportation to the nearest hospitals. As such, organs of nearly 400 people and their 800 kidneys and eyes go waste, buried or consigned to flames in funerals every day in India. Even if 50 of these kidneys are harvested per day, the problem of 'kidney scams' will vanish altogether, I believe.

The availability of legally harvested kidneys will stop the malpractice of illegal donations for money, exploitation of the poor and decrease the incentives fueling the kidney trade.

At present we do about 3,500 to 4,000 organ transplants a year in this country, out of which only a minuscule is cadaver transplants that really have a huge potential.

In the early seventies, I had spearheaded the concept that ONE LIFE SAVES FOUR LIVES. This is because in the process of transplanting two kidneys available from cadaver source, two dialysis machines are vacated for two patients in need of dialysis – thus one life lost in a fatal traffic accident can save four lives, two after transplantation and two upon receiving dialysis support.

Yet, fifty years later, I have to sadly admit that in India, in spite of our best efforts, the whole process of harvesting kidneys from traffic-donors has remained static. We don't have a dedicated air rescue service.

Had it succeeded, the programme would have eliminated the loopholes in the Indian Transplant Act, curbed the dirty kidney trade and exploitation of poor. It would have also brought down the high cost of transplantation and given a coat of white paint over the tarnished image of the country.

The quantum of stress, helplessness, and despair in failing to make cadaver kidney harvesting a success in the past 50 years has left me permanently scarred. The Transplant Act and all who participate in kidney transplantation from the beginning to end have no sympathy for the victim's suffering and the unparalleled pain and agony of the unrelated donor.

At the same time, it is a curse to suffer from irreversible kidney damage and not be rescued.

> **17 killed every hour in road mishaps in 2016**
>
> **Moushumi Das Gupta**
> moushumi.gupta@hindustantimes.com
>
> **NEW DELHI:** India witnessed 17 deaths and 55 road accidents every hour in 2016, one of the highest in the world, according to the latest report released by the Union road transport and highways ministry.
>
> ROAD ACCIDENTS KILLED 1,50,785 PEOPLE ACROSS THE COUNTRY IN 2016 – A 3.3% JUMP FROM 2015 WHEN 1,46,000 FATALITIES WERE REPORTED
>
> half or 46.3% of the road fatalities victim in 2016 were in the age-group of 18-35 years. The maximum number of road accidents — 1.9 lakh — occurred on two-lane roads. "Our target is to reduce the fatalities by 50% in next two years. The Motor Vehicle (Amendment) Bill pending in Parliament, if cleared in the next
>
> gone up by 10% during 2005-2015, road length during the same period increased only 3.75%. This has resulted in congestion on roads leading to a spike in accidents, experts said.
> The report shows drivers' fault was the single most important factor responsible for road accidents (84 per cent), killings

Iran has instituted a government-paid donors' scheme for a live donor for transplantation and has no shortage of kidneys with no reported malpractice and dialysis facilities in that country so far remain in surplus.

A similar attempt was made before in Chennai by Dr KC Reddy in the early nineties but unfortunately, it did not receive national acceptance – the concept of 'gifted' donation.

STOPPING THE TRADE STILL A CHALLENGE

In India, *the WHO-attributed 'altruistic (love and affection)' donation has become a loophole for illegal kidney trade.* Real donations of kidneys in the 'altruistic category' are negligible and in any case, exchange of gifts and other favourable gestures in kind, if not cash, are prevalent in most cases. Today, as of now, the commercialism in transplant business seem inevitable and any safeguards created is not yet fool proof.

HTEstates

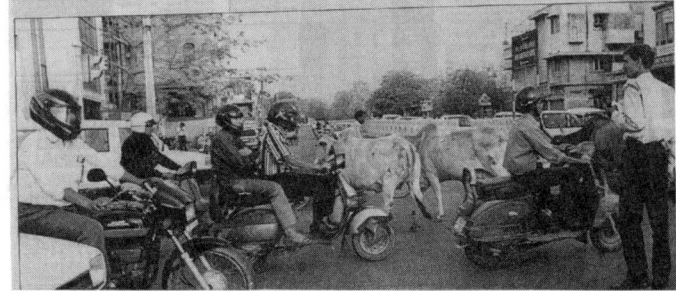

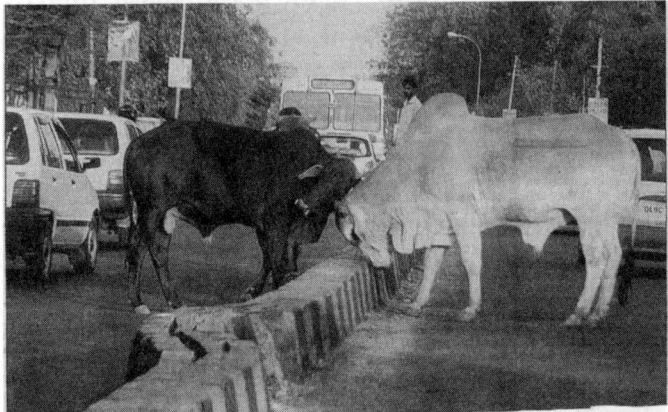

Battle at the line of control — Non-Legal – Human Fatality

MOVING FORWARD

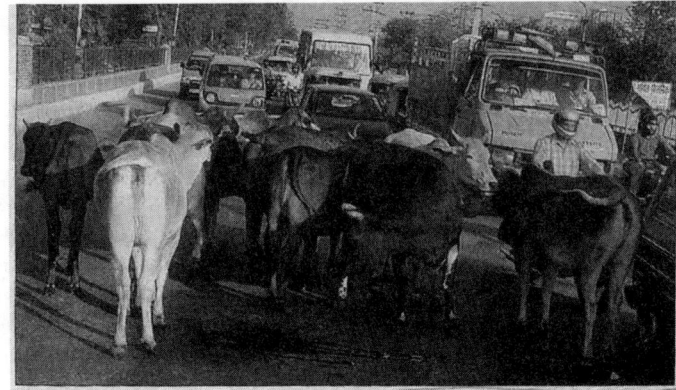

SANJEEV VERMA/HT
JUST ANOTHER DAY OUT: Stray cattle continue to create menace in the city. On Wednesday, a group of cows blocked Pankha Road near Janakpuri.

There are arguments in abundance suggesting 'if illegal markets are so exploitative why not legalise kidney trade for government regulation'?

The debate and following outcome of the 'Istanbul declaration' recommendations of the Amsterdam and Vancouver Forums[1] have not been able to contribute in minimising the unscrupulous trade of kidneys in India.

Our national associations have only described the magnitude of this complex problem of practice and trade of kidneys in India, not actually campaigned against it.

Cadaver kidney transplantation has remained confined to the kidneys harvested from brain dead patients in a hospital and distributed through National Organ & Tissue Transplant Organisation (NOTTO). There is little discussion on harvesting kidneys from fatal road traffic accidents in India.

For kidneys to be obtained from road traffic accidents, well-structured, government-approved guidelines would be required. It may appear a big task, but not impossible if there is a collective will to succeed – since India claims it is moving towards being the world's second largest economy.

---

[1] The Declaration of Istanbul was created at the Istanbul Summit on Organ Trafficking and Transplant Tourism held from 30 April to 1 May 2008 in Istanbul, Turkey.

The Declaration clarifies the issues of transplant tourism, trafficking and commercialism and provides ethical guidelines for practice in organ donation and transplantation. Since the creation of the declaration, over 100 countries have endorsed the principles. Some nations have subsequently strengthened their laws against commercial organ trade, including China, Israel, the Philippines, and Pakistan.

A National Organ Harvesting Programme (NOHP) can be formulated. The primary responsibility for formulating such a plan and programme is on the Union Ministry of Health. Such a country-wide programme must include an amendment in THOTA in which the participatory role of the State governments and law-keeping agencies is integrated in a very pro-active manner.[2] As of today police have no power to try THOTA cases, according to this piece of legislature.

After the first kidney transplant in Boston in 1953, we have just completed over seventy five years of this great achievement by pioneers, with ever-improving practice and progress, that has made kidney transplantation a routine clinical practice across the world.

However, worldwide, kidney transplantation continues to have a plethora of problems. Immunologic tissue reactions leading to Graft rejection with transplant nephropathy and calcineurin inhibitor toxicity and proteinuria are common still. Along with this is associated the recurrence of primary disease, emergence of hepatitis C and cytomegalic infections, BK Virus infection and susceptibility to bacterial infections. Besides the various infections is the problem of hypertension, hyper-lipidemia, bone and skin lesions, worsening cardio-vascular disease and emergence of other malignancies. The high cost of newer immunosuppressives, glucose intolerance and

---

[2] Reference: https://www.ncbi.nlm.nih.gov/pmc/articles/PMC3342642/

development of a diabetic state are added worries in case of a regular transplant.

As time passed, in India medical skills improved and with it kidney transplantations became popular. As the *demand* changed, the pattern of kidney donors changed from related to unrelated individuals. In the garb of being 'cousins', paid donors also changed the ratio of related to unrelated.

This single factor of 'demand and supply' was the overriding denominator in kidney transplantation in India until the turn of the century. In the '80s and '90s it resulted in a situation in which exploitation of the uneducated, uninformed and financially deprived donor became rampart. The incidences of high rate of transmission of infection including HIV, Hepatitis viruses and medical/surgical complications leading to morbidity and loss of graft by the recipients were unacceptably high. Yet demand for kidney transplants rose. In the absence of any authenticated information, however, no reliable data is available in this regard.

However, one thing has perceptibly changed. Money has now become the supreme denominator in this sector.

By the turn of the century, Bombay (Mumbai), Chennai, Calcutta (Kolkata), Bangalore, Hyderabad, Chandigarh and Delhi became the major centres for unrelated kidney transplantation in the country. Of course, the paucity of donors and ever rising demands have remained worldwide but lifelong economic burden continues to overshadow kidney transplantation in India.

ECONOMICS OF THE KIDNEY TRADE

At present times, the kidney trade in India has become extremely complicated, full of deceit and fraud at every level. It is a billion-dollar trade. Technology has helped the illegal trading practices and laws have not been able to keep up with the rapidly-changing nature of the crime.

Since easy transaction of cash and money are involved and possible – online transaction facilities helping to make dealers more faceless – the trade flourishes and remains under a complete shroud. Exchange of money is done at multiple levels and the entire control is in the hands of the 'boss' who is always invisible – a mafia boss, in other words.

TRANSACTION COST

The magnitude of the global kidney need can be gauged from a *Washington Post* report in 2016. It is said, in the beginning of that year, 100,791 patients in the United States needed and were waiting for a transplant. That year, 4,761 people died without transplant and only about 17,107 people managed to get a kidney transplant. A *US Today* report in August 2019 said, the United States discards about 3,500 donated kidneys a year, many of which could be used to save lives, new research shows.

The study, published in the journal *JAMA Internal Medicine*, focused on the rate at which donated kidneys were used in the US and France between 2004 and 2014. In that time, the US discarded about

17.9% of the kidneys it recovered, while France discarded about 9.1% of the kidneys it recovered. In all, the US threw away almost 28,000 donated kidneys in that 10-year period.

Nearly 100,000 Americans are on the waiting list for a kidney transplant, and about 12 people die each day waiting for a kidney transplant, this paper said. Meanwhile, about 10 kidneys are discarded daily, according to the National Kidney Foundation based in New York City. The study showed that kidneys discarded in the US were on average about 36 years old.[3]

This gives my readers a picture of the global need for kidneys and the world knows, India is where a kidney can be bought.[4]

The multiple workers such as middlemen and touts work at different levels but remain in communication with each other and the 'boss' and know how each step is to be micro-managed and has to be undertaken by all in the group. The whole practice of 'kidney donation' has become well-knit and undertaken by organised crime syndicates. Doctors are just one part of it.

Media reports say, 'India has about 100 renal transplant centres, of which 75% are with the private sector which has prohibitive costs. Every year about 2,500 to 3,000 renal transplants are done in India,

---

[3] https://www.usatoday.com/story/news/nation/2019/08/29/us-throws-away-3-500-donated-kidneys-per-year-study-says-heres-why/2139644001/

[4] https://www.washingtonpost.com/news/monkey-cage/wp/2016/12/07/organ-traffickers-lock-up-people-to-harvest-their-kidneys-here-are-the-politics-behind-the-organ-trade/?noredirect=on

of which only 100 are of cadaveric origin. About 50–60% of the kidneys for transplant come from 'unrelated living donors'.

The quantum of money involved for one transplant ranges of between ₹5 lakh to 20 lakh, depending upon the financial status, anxiety of recipient and health status of the patient.

For a patient coming from a distant part of the country and from neighbouring countries, the cost of a kidney is much higher.

The illegal trading is not about just demand and supply – as the demand will always be higher.

It is the *lust of the racketeer* who will prey on the poor, gullible and uneducated individuals and approach patients whose life is sustained on maintenance hemodialysis and have no matching kidney donors available. It is a well-knit syndicate of kingpins, middlemen, touts and paid field workers who are coherently involved at different levels under the close watch of each other.

The whole practice is based upon the 'rich and poor' divide that operates in India's social milieu. In my over fifty years of working in this field of kidney transplantation, I have still to see an educated and financially solvent individual coming forward to donate a kidney to a poorer individual in his/her family circle just out of *altruism* – leave aside to an 'unrelated' known patient on maintenance hemodialysis.

There are no details available of this nature even in cadaveric transplantation.

REALITY CHECK

In the new centres where the practice of transplantation is of optimally high standard, the number of neglected transplant cases has reduced significantly. The deterrents resulting from the Transplantation of Human Organs Act, 1994 (THOA) promulgated by the Government of India have reduced open uncontrolled transplant activity.

Today, there is better selection of the 'living unrelated donor' who is HLA matched. The fever and post-operative complications are better managed and with effective and upgraded immunosuppressive regimen, the total outcome has remarkably improved. But the malpractices of the trade of kidney remains a stigma on this country despite the Act (THOTA) and kidney scandals and scams are recurrently seen.

In present times of rapid technological advance, misuse of these same technologies is rampant and the name, address, aadhaar card, voter I-card and any other documents required are falsified and fictitiously created to meet the recipient-donor-hospital requirements. All that one needs is a software operator.

A poor kidney donor is always manipulated and there is no will to take care of the donor, either on the part of the recipient nor the hospital involved. Both, hospitals and relatives of the recipients, just do not consider care of the live donor an important aspect of kidney transplantation. There are no binding regulations for such post-hospital discharge care of a kidney donor. The paid kidney donors are subjected to inhumane neglect by families of recipients, doctors and hospitals as nobody wants to know them anymore.

Their humiliation and neglect include insufficient payments, poor health care and to an extent, the law-keeping agencies too treat them shabbily. In India, 'paisa liya' – you have accepted money – is a socially looked-down upon practice. Unfortunately, and painfully, there are no follow-ups of an 'unrelated paid kidney donor' in any hospital in the country.

In a study of 'follow-ups' – in a social investigation research in Chennai in 2002 – 300 paid donors were interviewed. As many as 95% of these donors told the investigators they had 'donated for money' and the money received was far less than the promised amount.[5]

---

[5] Dr Lawrence Cohen has done extensive studies in India regarding organ trafficking.

Interactions of experts with kidney recipients from India revealed that not only the sellers but also the buyers are at risk.

Having spent a large amount of money on buying a kidney and the transplant procedure, many of them are not able to sustain the long-term immunosuppressant therapy which is necessary to prevent rejection of the transplant by the recipients' body. Often, they underestimate the long-term costs and their monthly income cannot sustain these unanticipated expenses, which results in kidney failure.

In addition to this, there is also the problem of the younger generation of nephrologists going ahead with transplantation surgeries without doing sufficient tissue factor matches. This again results in the need to take immunosuppressant therapy for longer periods. It is also observed that in the long run, more than the kidney buyer (in addition to the brokers, the doctors and the transplant centres), the drug companies benefit substantially from the whole process.

(Fr Mathew Abraham CSsR, Health Secretary, Catholic Bishops' Conference of India. Paper presented at The Pontifical Academy of Social

The study showed that as many as 75% continued to live in debts, 90% had poorer health and 30% of the wives were *forced to donate* to meet husband's money requirements.

All donations were channeled through middlemen and organised syndicates. Over 80% of these very donors today advocate against paid donations. Similar results have been recognised in 'commercial trading of organs' in Iran (Targooshi, 2002).

The stark fact is, that the poor who is deprived, uneducated and always in need of finances, remains at the end of supply line and often gets nothing in his/her life.

Doctors are often accused of callousness and advancing their own financial gains, who exploit fellow humans in pain and with health problems. At the same time, in our country they are placed at par with God. In this process, the Doctor becomes a tool in the hands of his patients and his family and others in the society. The cases of 'Kidney Rackets' involving acclaimed and senior kidney physicians in the country need a final solution, both for the doctors and the exploited poor.

Clearly, paid transplantation is not the solution for this mode of treatment worldwide.

It is more *not right* in a country like India where 'legal licensing' of any activity becomes a 'legal protection of malpractice' and exploitation by the

---

Sciences -*Human Trafficking: Issues Beyond* 17 – 21 April, 2015 Casina Pio IV, Vatican City.)
   http://www.endslavery.va/content/endslavery/en/publications/acta_20/abraham.html

middleman – be it in construction, prohibition, prostitution or transplantation.

Then we begin to call it 'Corruption'. The large population, lack of education, economic deprivation and overall 'the middleman' present at the individual or syndicate levels prevail over these various commercial activities.

NEED TO MODIFY THOTA, 2014

As our country tops in the world in road traffic accidents – harvesting of kidneys from these unfortunate victims is the only solution to the shortage of kidneys for transplantation in our country.

We need modification of the Transplantation Act to harvest kidneys and other organs from fatal road traffic accidents rather than letting such organs rot in mortuaries, be buried or consigned to flames in cremations. On the roads across the whole country no *middlemen* or *cousins* operate yet. No malpractices or intentional traffic accidents occur yet. Accident victims are still rushed to Emergency and Trauma Care facilities where regular doctors try to save lives. If not, provisions in law should provide for waning lives to contribute to saving other lives.

There is, therefore, an urgent need to recognise and exploit this rather unfortunate source of organ harvesting. The ethics and practice of transplantation will then get a chance to remain clean and the suffering, economic burden and chaos for the 'donor' will not happen as there will be no live donor, except relatives mostly.

I call it 'Instant Cadaver Transplantation' – howsoever grim the reality is.

It is the loss of life on roads which can give life and hope to the dying in hospitals and homes in India. *The awareness of organ donation from cadaver source is of paramount importance in this country – more so in India* than elsewhere in the world. One does wish there are more people like actor and sportsperson Rahul Bose who has pledged 'every part' of his body for organ donation.[6]

---

[6] http://www.newindianexpress.com/entertainment/hindi/2019/sep/20/rahul-bose-to-pledge-for-organ-donation-after-death-2036552.html

THE AWARDS AND ACCOLADES

The Government of India has been giving the Padma awards in recognition of pioneering work in the field of Nephrology and Kidney Transplantation to caregivers and surgeons practicing in this sector since the 1980s. Among them are:

Dr RVS Yadav   Padma Shri 1982
    Kidney Transplant Surgeon
    (New Delhi)

Dr Muthu Krishna Mani   Padma Bhushan 1991
    (Chennai)

Dr Ramesh Kumar   Padma Shri 1992
    (New Delhi)   Padma Bhushan 2003

Dr Kirpal Singh Chugh   Padma Shri 2000
    (Chandigarh)

Dr DS Rana   Padma Shri 2009
    (New Delhi)

Dr Anil Kumar Bhalla   Padma Shri 2010
    (New Delhi)

Dr Sarbeswar Sahariah   Padma Shri 2014
    Kidney Transplant Surgeon
    (Hyderabad)

Dr Hargovind Laxmishankar   Padma Shri 2015
    Trivedi
    (Ahmedabad)

Dr Mukut Minz   Padma Shri 2017
   Kidney Transplant Surgeon
   (Chandigarh)

Dr Sandeep Guleria   Padma Shri 2019
   2019 (New Delhi)

EPILOGUE

I have spent my entire life in creating treatments for kidney diseases and furthering treatment modalities for a vast number of patients suffering from kidney ailments. I have myself lost count of the cures and failures in my professional life. But one failure hurts me. The failure to contain trading and commercialisation of kidney transplants in my own country.

Today, life-style illnesses and diabetic kidney diseases have taken precedence over all other diseases effecting kidneys. There is no end in sight for this hurricane of a problem and has resulted in poor health profile of the average individual and a plethora of diseases affecting the common Indian in our country. Chronic kidney disease has become a major health problem which requires immediate creation of dialysis facilities and kidney transplantation across the nation. At the same time, just three months ago, in June 2019 a top Delhi hospital CEO was arrested for malpractice.[1] Rumour is even now rife in Delhi's slum colonies close to corporate

---

[1] https://timesofindia.indiatimes.com/city/kanpur/international-kidney-racket-busted-in-kanpur-delhi-psri-hospital-ceo-taken-into-custody-for-questioning/articleshow/69701554.cms

hospitals that missing children have been kidnapped by organ traders. Even as I conclude my book, the doctor in news is a young urologist, pleading for assistance for his dialysis patients.[2] And there is hope in the news of attempts to generate organs from the dead.[3]

The ideal solution to chronic kidney failure is transplantation and there is always widening gap between demand and availability of kidney donors. Inevitably, there is malpractice, exploitation of the poor and gullible where unscrupulous individuals are deeply involved in the kidney trade.

The Transplantation Act is extremely stringent, yet kidney scandals are rampant. And if you follow the media reports, one cannot but notice that the same 'kingpin', the same set of individuals making up a gang, the same suspected doctors keep surfacing again and again – only the city is different, hospital is different, the donor is different and the recipient. The modality of operation remains the same, the doctors just change hospitals in which they are employed. One must also mention here, conviction is low – the speed of trial snaillike, the casework poor, police often paid to muddle the paperwork or keep it pending and courts are not educated on the social impact, health impact of the scandals and scams in

---

[2] https://thewire.in/health/kashmiri-doctor-medical-concerns-police
[3] https://bigthink.com/surprising-science/dead-bodies-move
   https://www.sciencedirect.com/science/article/pii/S2589871X19301421
   https://bigthink.com/stephen-johnson/scientists-successfully-reanimate-the-brains-of-decapitated-pigs

organ trade – they just look at points of law which more often than not allows culprits to get away. Even the bail facilities and jurisdiction to try and award punishment need an urgent re-look in case of kidney trade charges.

The ideal kidney donor is the victim of fatal traffic accidents on the roads in our country. India's vehicular movement is second to China and in fatal accidents India tops in the chart. I see no other alternative except to harvest kidneys from unfortunate victims on the road. One life lost will save four lives resulting in two kidney transplants and ready availability of two hemodialysis machines. My last words in this book is: We – the medical fraternity and hospital authorities – and the government/s must resolve together to put this action plan in motion. All nations in the world do it this way. Then, why not us Indians? Why can't we change this tarnished national image?

APPENDIX A

The Transplantation of Human Organs (Amendment) Act, 2011.

On 27th September 2011, the Act of 1994 was amended primarily for prevention of continuing commercial dealings in human organs.

The principal components of these amendments were:

a. Amendment of section 2, subsection (hb) 'minor' means a person who has not completed the age of eighteen years.
b. Amendment of section 2, subsection (b) for clause (i) 'near relative' means a spouse, son, daughter, father, mother, brother, sister, grandfather, grandmother, grandson or granddaughter.
c. Provision of a transplant coordinator in each hospital conducting transplantation.
d. Enlargement of advisory committees to advise appropriate authority and inclusions of one administrative expert in the name of secretary of the State government, two medical experts, joint director of Ministry of Health and department of welfare, two eminent social workers and one

legal expert, one person from non-government organisation working in the field of organ donations or human rights and lastly one specialist in the field of human organ transplantation, not a member of the transplant team.
e. Revised amendments for punishments for illegal dealings in human tissues.
f. Establishment of National or Regional or State Human Organs and Tissue removal and storage networks.

Establishment of National Registry regarding donors and recipients of human organ and tissues.

The Transplantation of Human Organs and Tissues Act, 1994, as amended in 2011 was further modified and various loopholes were plugged. This final blueprint of Transplant of Human Organs and Tissues Rules, 2014 is the present-day 'Bible' which governs all transplantation activity in India.

The Transplantation of Human Organs and Tissues Rules, 2014 stipulates:

Rule 7, sub-rule (3) when the proposed donor and the recipient are not near relatives

(i) There is no commercial transaction between the recipient and the donor and that no payment has been made to the donor or promised to be made to the donor or any other person;

(ii) An explanation of the link between them and the circumstances which led to the offer being made;

(iii) The reasons why the donor wishes to donate;
(iv) The documentary evidence of the link, e.g. proof that they have lived together, etc.;
(v) Old photographs showing the donor and the recipient together;
(vi) There is no middleman or tout involved;
(vii) Financial status of the donor and the recipient to give appropriate evidence of their vocation and income for the previous three financial years and any gross disparity between the status of the two;
(viii) The donor is not a drug addict;
(ix) The near relative or if near relative is not available, any adult person related to donor by blood or marriage of the proposed unrelated donor is interviewed regarding awareness about his or her intension to donate and the reasons for donation, and any strong views or disagreement or objection of such kin.

Rule 7, sub-rule (4) In case of swap donation referred to under subsection (3A) of section 9 of the Act shall be approved by Authorisation Committee of hospital or district or State in which transplantation is proposed to be done and the donation of organs shall be permissible only from near-relatives of the swap recipients.

Rule 7, sub-rule (5) When the recipient is in a critical condition in need of life saving organ transplantation within a week, the donor or recipient may approach hospital incharge to expedite evaluation by the Authorisation Committee.

Rule 20. Procedure in case of foreigners: When the proposed donor or the recipient are foreigners:

(a) A senior Embassy official of the country of origin has to certify the relationship between the donor and the recipient as per Form 21 and in case a country does not have an Embassy in India, the certificate of relationship, in the same format, shall be issued by the Government of that country.

(b) The Authorisation Committee shall examine the cases of all Indian donors consenting to donate organs to a foreign national (who is a near relative), including a foreign national of Indian origin, with greater caution and such cases should be considered rarely on case to case basis.

(c) The Indian living donors wanting to donate to a foreigner other than near relative shall not be considered.

Rule 22. Precautions in case of woman donor: Greater precautions ought to be taken and her identity and independent consent should be confirmed by a person other than the recipient.

KIDNEY TRANSPLANTATION IN INDIA
OFFENCES AND PENALTIES

(The Transplantation of Human Organs and Tissues Act, 2014)

Section 18. Punishment for removal of human organs or tissues or both without authority.

(1) Any person who renders his services to or at any hospital and who, for purposes of transplantation, conducts, associates with, or helps in any manner in, the removal of any human organ without authority, shall be punishable with imprisonment for a term which may extend to ten years and with fine which may extend to twenty lakh rupees.

(2) Where any person convicted under sub-section (1) is a registered medical practitioner, his name shall be reported by the Appropriate Authority to the respective State Medical Council for taking necessary action including the removal of his name from the register of the Council for a period of three years for the first offence and permanently for the subsequent offence.

(3) Any person who renders his services to or at any hospital and who conducts, or associates with or helps in any manner in the removal of human tissues without authority, shall be punishable with imprisonment for a term which may extend to three years and with fine which may extend to five lakh rupees.

Section 19. Punishment for commercial dealings in human tissues – Whoever:

(a) Makes or receives any payment for the supply of, or for an offer to supply, any human tissue; or
(b) Seeks to find person willing to supply for payment and human tissue; or
(c) Offers to supply any human tissue for payment; or

(d) Initiates or negotiates any arrangements involving the making of any payment for the supply of, or for an offer to supply, any human organ;

(e) Takes part in the management or control of a body of persons, whether a society, firm or company, whose activities consist of or include the initiation or negotiation of any arrangement;

(f) Publishes or distributes or causes to be published or distributed any advertisement:

   (i) Inviting persons to supply for payment of any human organ;
   (ii) Offering to supply any human organ for payment; or
   (iii) Indicating that the advertiser is willing to initiate or negotiate any arrangement referred to in clause (d);

(g) Abets in the preparation or submission of false documents including giving false affidavits to establish that the donor is making the donation of the human organs, as a near relative or by reason of affection or attachment towards the recipient, shall be punishable with imprisonment for a term which shall not be less than five years but which may extend to ten years and shall be liable to fine which shall not be less than twenty lakh rupees but which may extend to one crore rupees.

Section 19A. Punishment for illegal dealing in human tissues.

Section 20. Punishment for contravention of any other provision of this Act.

Section 21. Offences by companies.

Section 22. Cognizance of offence.

Section 23. Protection of action taken in good faith (Altruistic).

(1) No suit, prosecution or other legal proceeding shall lie against any person for anything which is in good faith done or intended to be done in pursuance of the provisions of this Act.
(2) No suit or other legal proceeding shall lie against the Central Government or the State Government for any damage caused or likely to be caused for anything which is in good faith done or intended to be done in pursuance of the provisions of this Act.

Guidelines issued by Directorate General of Health Services, Delhi-110032 on 10.4.2017.

1. Documents of each transplant patient to be thoroughly scrutinized and signed by the legal cell and the transplant cell of the hospital before presenting the same to the committee for approval of transplantation.
2. In case of spousal donor, 'Marriage Registration Certificate' is insisted upon to be as a proof. The Certificate may be got verified by sending the same via post/speed post to the issuing authority.
3. Aadhaar Card should be verified online and screen shot of same should be maintained the file.

4. Donor and the recipient should be asked to provide old family photographs of association (minimum 2 nos) to verify genuineness of the relationship. HLA/DNA typing of the parents / children may be done, if required.
5. In case of international patients, vigil should be kept avoiding accepting forged documents (Passport) unknowingly.
6. **Form 20** issued by the Tehsildar must also be got verified by speedpost.
7. Some mechanism should be in place to detect Photoshop.
8. In case of foreigners, **Form 21** from the embassy should be collected by the designated hospital staff. It should not be left to patients or relatives. Its issue by the respective embassy be got verified through official mail.
9. Photo ID proof must be enclosed in the file of the person giving consent to the donor.
10. All originals are to be produced before the committee in the meetings.
11. A mechanism to keep a check on the supporting staff who are involved in preparing the cases of transplant be put in place.
12. Meetings are to be conducted within closed doors and video graphed.
13. Good-quality audio and video equipments should be used for audio-visual recordings.
14. ID of interpreter/translator should be placed in the file. As far as possible interpreter employed by the hospital or professional interpreter not related to donor/recipient be engaged.

15. Minutes of each authorisation committee meeting is to be issued in prescribed name and put on portal of the hospital.
16. SOPs of the file movement till approval or rejection are to be prepared and circulated by the hospital/MS. In case of rejection, the patient must be informed via speaking order.
17. It may be ensured that files are provided to members at least one day before the Authorisation Committee meeting.
18. Details of income of recipient and donor for the last three years including ITR, bank details/statements etc. should be placed in the file.
19. Details of the funding agency/NGO (if any) should be placed in the file.
20. All pages in the files for authorisation committee should be numbered.
21. A group may be created using email ID's/Phone numbers / Whatsapp for easy and effective communication.

APPENDIX B

NOTTO – NATIONAL ORGAN AND TISSUE TRANSPLANT ORGANISATION

The National Organ and Tissue Transplant Organisation (NOTTO) is a national-level organisation set up under the Directorate General of Health Services, Ministry of Health and Family Welfare, Government of India. It has two divisions: the 'National Human Organ and Tissue Removal and Storage Network' and the 'National Biomaterial Centre'.

THE LEGISLATION IS AS FOLLOWS

National Human Organ and Tissue Removal and Storage Network.

This has been mandated as per the Transplantation of Human Organs (Amendment) Act 2011. The network will be established initially for Delhi and gradually expanded to include other States and Regions of the country. This division of the NOTTO is the nodal networking agency for Delhi and shall network for Procurement, Allocation and Distribution of Organs and Tissues in Delhi.

FUNCTION/ACTIVITIES

National Network division of NOTTO would function as apex centre for All India activities of coordination and networking for procurement and distribution of Organs and Tissues and registry of Organs and Tissues Donation and Transplantation in the country. The following activities would be undertaken to facilitate Organ Transplantation in the safest way in shortest possible time and *to collect data to develop and publish a National registry:*

At National Level:
- Lay down policy guidelines and protocols for various functions.
    - Network with similar regional and State-level organisations.
    - All registry data from States and Regions would be compiled and published.
    - Creating awareness, promotion of organ donation and transplantation activities.
    - Co-ordination from procurement of organs and tissues to transplantation when organ is allocated outside the region.
    - Dissemination of information to all concerned organisations, hospitals and individuals.
    - Monitoring of transplantation activities in the Regions and States and maintaining databank in this regard.
    - To assist in data management for organ transplant surveillance and organ transplant and Organ Donor registry.

APPENDIX B

- o Consultancy support on the legal and non-legal aspects of donation and transplantation.
- o Coordinate and Organise trainings for various cadre of workers.

For Delhi and NCR
- Maintaining the waiting list of terminally ill patients requiring transplants.
    - o Networking with transplant centres, retrieval centres and tissue banks.
    - o Co-ordination for all activities required for procurement of organs and tissues including medico legal aspects.
    - o Matching of recipients with donors.
    - o Allocation, Transportation, Storage and Distribution of Organs and Tissues within Delhi and National Capital Territory region.
    - o Post-transplant patients and living donor follow-up for assessment of graft rejection, survival rates etc.
    - o Awareness, Advocacy and Training workshops and other activities for promotion of organ donation.

APPENDIX C

A contributory, shared fund for people for healthcare was BR Ambedkar's idea.

The **ESI** scheme is a government supported scheme known as the Employees State Insurance Scheme, enacted in 1948. This Act and its guidelines provide for insurance entitlement to which the government as well as the employer and employee contribute a sum that is made available to an employee at times of certain kind of needs. The government has a budget of about ₹1,500 crore for this. (https://www.esic.nic.in/attachments/publicationfile/c359b08d8d4ca07bb35f9734f88c530c.pdf.)

ESI is applicable to all factories and other establishments as defined in the Act with 10 or more persons employed in such an establishment and the beneficiaries' monthly wage does not exceed ₹21,000. Only such persons are covered under the scheme. As of July 2019, it covers about 3.6 crore government employees. Since 2011 it has been extended to shops, hotels, restaurants, private medical and educational institutions, cinemas and newspaper establishments employing 20 or more persons.

The ESI benefits include medical, cash, maternity, disability and dependent benefits to the Insured

APPENDIX C

Persons under the ESI Act. The contributions made by the employee and the employer fund these ESI benefits. Since July 2019, the employers' contribution has been reduced to 3.25 per cent of the fund and employees' contribution has been reduced to 0.75 per cent. The scheme is supposed to provides full medical care to the employee registered under the ESI Act, 1948 during the period of his incapacity, restoration of his health and working capacity. It is supposed to provide financial assistance to compensate for the loss of wages during the period of his abstention from work due to sickness, maternity and employment injury and during the hospitalisation cost in any ESI hospital. The scheme is supposed to provide medical care to the employee family members also. (https://www.financialexpress.com/money/insurance/esi-act-applicability-benefits-eligibility-and-new-contribution-rates-from-july-1/1607435/) The disbursing authority is the Employees' State Insurance Corporation, a statutory body under the care of the Ministry of Labour and Employment, Government of India. Outpatient medical facilities are available in 1,418 ESI dispensaries and through 1,678 registered medical practitioners. Inpatient care is available in 145 ESI hospitals and 42 hospital annexes with a total of 19,387 beds. In addition, several State government hospitals also have beds for the exclusive use of ESI Beneficiaries. Cash benefits can be availed in any of 830 ESI centres throughout India.

The Ex-servicemen Contributory Health Scheme or **ECHS** is a flagship scheme of the Ministry of

Defence, Department of Ex-Servicemen Welfare. The aim of this scheme is to provide quality healthcare to Ex-servicemen pensioners and their dependents. As on 1 May 2015, a total of 1,521,563 Ex-servicemen have enlisted with the scheme along with 3,202,610 dependents.

The service has one central headquarter centre in Delhi and 28 regional centres with 426 polyclinics throughout the country (as of 2015 data http://www.desw.gov.in/ex-servicemen-contributory-health-scheme/about-echs).

For 2019–2020, the ECHS had projected a requirement of about ₹6,000 crore, but was given only about ₹3,200 crore, almost the same as the previous year. To avoid strain on its resources, the Army has asked the Defence Ministry to remove the allocation for the Ex-Servicemen Contributory Health Scheme (ECHS) from its budget and move it under the defence pension fund, which is a separate entity within the defence budget. (https://economictimes.indiatimes.com/articleshow/70729023.cms?from=mdr&utm_source=contentofinterest&utm_medium=text&utm_campaign=cppst)

So, for the healthcare needs of about five crore people including ex-soldiers, the government has about ₹5000 crore earmarked in a year. If any of these beneficiaries develop kidney trouble, they are provided primary-level care in the ECHS and ESI centres. After a point, needing end-stage care, ESI patients are told to go to private hospitals and bear the costs of kidney care themselves.

APPENDIX C

No ESI patient has ever been paid for a kidney transplant so far.

Despite all the brouhaha about the armed forces in India, even ex-servicemen are rendered helpless at the cost of private care for kidney-related services, including dialysis and catheter services. Even in ECHS cases, kidney transplant, of course, is an expensive proposition in any army hospital.

ACKNOWLEDGEMENTS

Though I had been watching the march of India's kidney bazaars, kidney trade and kidney scandals since mid-1970s and collecting newspaper and magazine articles, inadvertently, when I became a victim of such a scandal in my own department, designated a centre of excellence, at Batra Hospital in May 2017 – I got thinking.

This involvement of a hospital I had been associated with for three decades was a grievous injury to my unblemished professional standing of almost half a century. I am a care giver. It is my paid job and my profession. It took many months of deep introspection for me to actually realise the importance of this whole virulent saga and that if I, the senior-most of the country's leading nephrologists, did not do something about it, I would be remiss in my duty to my profession.

I eventually decided to publish the whole story of this socio-medical malady in India. At this stage my secretary in the department, Samarjit Singh started spending hours with me, exploring all of what was available in the world on this subject. He did it with admirable interest and spend a whole year doing so. I remain extremely thankful to him.

ACKNOWLEDGEMENTS

Both of us are totally novice and amateurs in this challenging task of aggregating the entire information collected at this stage. Later Mary D'Souza helped in preparing the final draft.

I also take this opportunity to acknowledge all the media houses from where I have used references, clippings, images in the public domain. I also acknowledge Creative Commons information from Wikipedia and Wikimedia.

We had no idea of how to approach acclaimed publishers in Delhi and sent letters to twenty such addresses. I was overwhelmed with eleven positive responses from publishing houses. I thank them all.

I thank Naveen Chawla, former Election Commissioner of India, for giving a Foreword to the book, championing my cause, despite his many engagements and busy schedule. I also thank Justice Sudershan Misra for his appreciation of my work.

I first talked to Renu Kaul Verma, Managing Director of Vitasta Publishing Private Limited. We clicked at first conversation. We soon had a meeting at the India International Centre, and I was highly impressed with her friendly and caring approach towards a professional with a raw manuscript for publication as a book. I do not know if she had noticed my passion and my commitment to find a solution to eradicate the socio-medical crime that encompasses kidney transplantation. She encouraged me and accepted this proposal by me in our first meeting. Since then there has been a very helpful approach by her all throughout and I remain indebted to her.

I thank her profusely for extending all help to this green-horn writer like me.

Papri Sri Raman, a veteran journalist and Publishing Director of Vitasta Publishing House, was requested to personally undertake the arduous task of turning into a readable book a raw manuscript that I had to offer. Before thanking her, I wish to admire her profile of a prolific and meticulous writer-editor. I met her first at Vitasta headquarters and remember her deep and professional conversation with me regarding the purpose and projection of this 'never written before' subject of kidney bazaars and trade in India. She educated me on various aspects of this book and its process. The presentation of this book is entirely her brainchild. She has painstakingly edited each word and line of the manuscript in a professional fashion. I remain indebted and deeply thankful to her for her immense help.

I thank Renu and Papri's editorial team including Suhani Adhar, and marketing team – all due to my choosing Vitasta. I have followed each notification of Vitasta Publications on Twitter and other social media platforms and feel fortunate in my de novo attempt at professional writing. I have no long innings to write many books – except a couple more with the help of this publishing house and I remain hopeful.

I know that SAGE is a publishing house of international repute and I thank them and their technical and marketing staff for partnering Vitasta in bringing to the public domain my book. I am indebted to Aarti David for motivating me to go with Sage on its own merit. She has personally followed

ACKNOW-LEDGEMENTS

the progress of this work and not to forget the sterling assistance from Manisha and Savitha along with Papri who have collectively streamlined the production.

I acknowledge my emotional gratitude to my granddaughter Ashna who spent long hours editing my initial writeups during my short visits to Dallas, USA. In the process I discovered that she is on the editorial board of her university and is a prolific writer herself. She is now completing her graduation course and our mutual affinity is an open secret in our family. I feel singularly blessed.

My elder son Sumit, an accomplished and acclaimed nephrologist who is director of Texus Kidney Institute in Dallas, was highly appreciative of my effort to stem the kidney trade in India to begin with but later was apprehensive about writing the manuscript on such a sensitive subject in this country. As months passed by, he however, constantly encouraged me and remained in the loop of my writings. He has once again visited me now and was able to go through the manuscript and said, 'Daddy I am proud of you'. His endorsement became an extremely satisfying event in my family and I feel grateful to him and others in my own lifetime.

My second son Nishant, an executive in NTT Data, formerly Dell, had expressed his apprehension in publishing a book on such a troublesome subject in India. I had appraised him that these writings are my forty years' observation of the medico-social malady in the country and carried no motive at all. He has supported me throughout despite his apprehensions and has remained abreast of the progress of the manuscript. I have felt the importance of such a support in the family and I remain thankful to him.

Last but not the least, I thank my wife Kalpana for supporting me during my formative years as a specialist doctor, alone, innocently and solidly. She has been the cornerstone of my long professional march of more than 50 years. At times, she reminds me of this fact, and, of course, takes pride singularly. I thank Kalpana for all good thing in our life together and for standing tall and firm regarding this book.

ABOUT THE AUTHOR

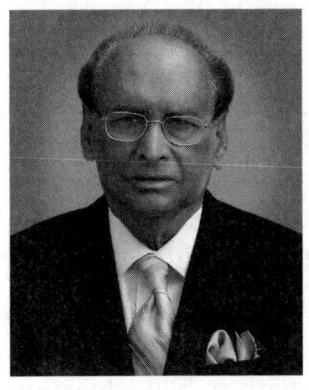

Dr Ramesh Kumar is a pioneer in the field of Nephrology (kidney diseases) in India and South East Asia. Nephrology has grown with him in the country.

Born on 16 June 1940 at Khurja, Bulandshahr, Uttar Pradesh, he did his Doctor in Medicine (MD) from Agra University and was rated as the 'Best Overseas Young Physician' while training in Nephrology at Queens University, Belfast and later at Charing Cross Hospital, London. He obtained the degree of MRCP in renal diseases and medicine in 1971.

He was elected fellow (FRCP) at the Royal College of Physicians, Edinburgh in 1981 for his pioneering contributions in establishing and furtherance of dialysis and kidney transplantation in India.

Beginning at All India Medical Institute (AIIMS) in 1972, in a career span of nearly fifty years, Ramesh Kumar has the clear distinction of starting the

ABOUT THE AUTHOR

artificial kidney programme including kidney transplantation in Northern India. As a pioneer of CAPD, he made available an alternative mode of dialysis treatment. He identified patterns of kidney diseases in India and established training programmes for medical, technical and nursing staff in Nephrology countrywide. He has been the guiding force in creation of dialysis centres across Northern India.

Following his relentless crusade of 20 years, the Transplantation of Human Organ Act was passed by Parliament in May 1994. With enactment of the Transplantation Act, the open organ trading has stopped but is continuing in a clandestine manner and kidney scams surface with impunity periodically across the whole nation. Dr Ramesh Kumar is deeply concerned and has made a bold effort in highlighting the malady in his book.

His endeavours continue with public education programmes for kidney diseases and in showcasing India abroad as a centre of excellence for world kidney care.

He is the recipient of multiple awards and accolades and recipient of numerous international fellowships, visiting professorships and is guest speaker worldwide.

Dr Ramesh Kumar has been Chief Physician to former Prime Minister Atal Bihari Vajpayee, several Health Ministers and many other leaders in the country.

He was awarded Padma Shri in 1992 and Padma Bhushan in 2003.

Let this book be your companion and guide as you try to make sense of the forthcoming tumultuous events in Indian politics.

Lord Meghnad Desai
Economist, Author and Politician

A political tale of India through the first-person narratives of political leaders

For special offers on this and other books from SAGE, write to marketing@sagepub.in

Explore our range at **www.sagepub.in**

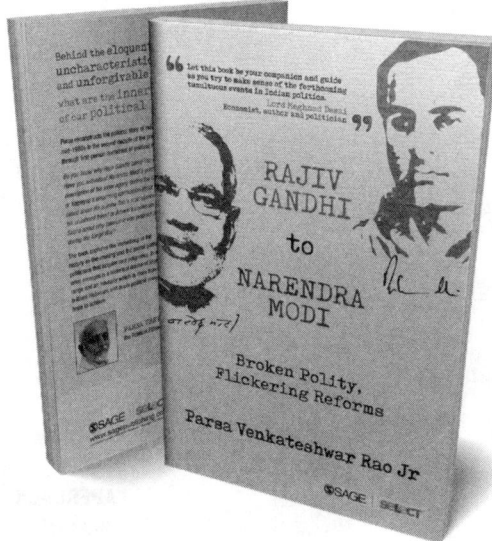

PAPERBACK
9789353282981

> It's great to see a book capturing the magical journey of Indian football being written. I wish *India's Football Dream* and its authors Mr Shantanu Gupta and Mr Nikhil Sharma the very best, and hope it serves as a tool to educate every Indian about the 'beautiful game' in our country.
>
> **Praful Patel**
> *President, All India Football Federation*

A book about how Football has grown as one of the most loved sports in India

For special offers on this and other books from SAGE, write to marketing@sagepub.in

Explore our range at www.sagepub.in

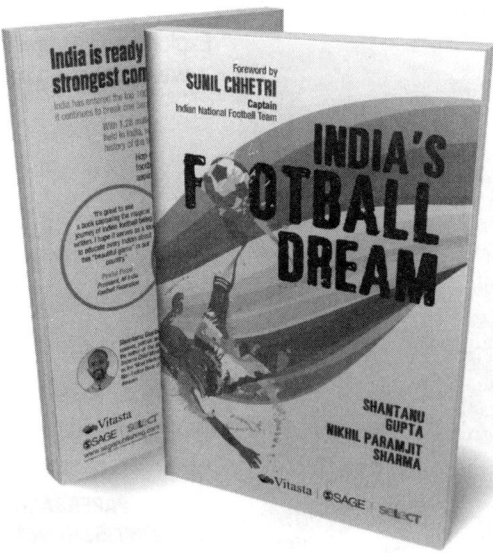

PAPERBACK
9789353283056

Professor Ramachandran's learned, insightful and fascinating book on Hinduism, marked by his original views and strong opinions, makes for a stimulating and instructive reading.

Shashi Tharoor

The history of Hinduism from Rigvedic times to the present and an analysis of its future in India

For special offers on this and other books from SAGE, write to marketing@sagepub.in

Explore our range at www.sagepub.in

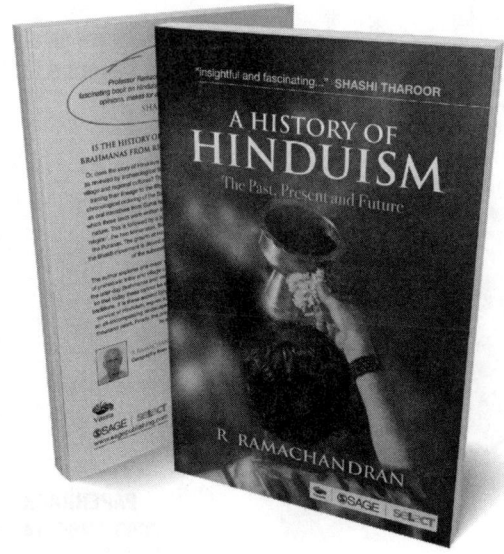

PAPERBACK
9789352806980

> I see this book coming at a very interesting time—it focuses on hope and optimism rather than worrying about the world. It focuses on how the world will, could and has always come together to serve its own people.
>
> **Dr Purvi Mehta**
> *Head of Asia Agriculture, Bill and Melinda Gates Foundation*

The joy of giving!

For special offers on this and other books from SAGE, write to marketing@sagepub.in

Explore our range at
www.sagepub.in

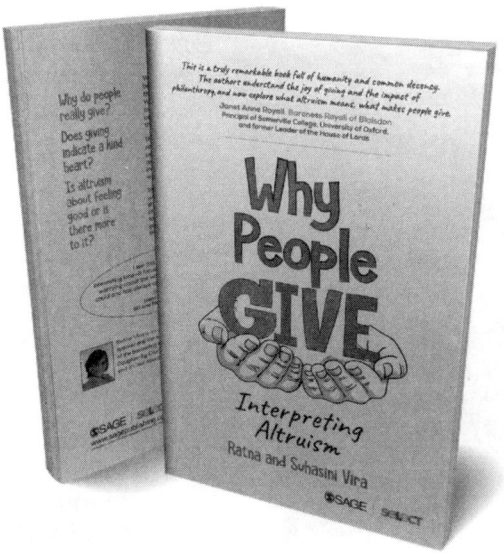

PAPERBACK
9789353285814